25 Natural Ways
to Relieve
Irritable Bowel Syndrome

Also by James Scala, Ph.D.

Arthritis: Diet Against It
The High Blood Pressure Relief Diet
If You Can't/Won't Stop Smoking
Making the Vitamin Connection
The New Arthritis Relief Diet
The New Eating Right for a Bad Gut
Prescription for Longevity
25 Natural Ways to Relieve Stress and Prevent Burnout

25 Natural Ways
to Relieve
Irritable Bowel Syndrome

A MIND-BODY APPROACH TO WELL-BEING

James Scala, Ph.D.

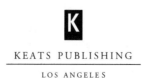

KEATS PUBLISHING

LOS ANGELES

NTC/Contemporary Publishing Group

Library of Congress Cataloging-in-Publication Data

Scala, James, 1934–
      25 natural ways to relieve irritable bowel syndrome : a mind-body approach to well-being / James Scala.
         p. cm.
      Includes index.
      ISBN 0-658-00701-7
      1. Irritable colon-Alternative treatment—Popular works. 2. Colon (Anatomy)—Diseases—Popular works. 3. Irritable colon—Popular works. I. Title: Twenty-five natural ways to relieve irritable bowel syndrome. II. Title.

      RC862.177 S27 2000
      616.3'42-dc21   00-063036

Published by Lowell House
A division of NTC/Contemporary Publishing Group, Inc.
4255 West Touhy Avenue, Lincolnwood, Illinois 60712, U.S.A.

Managing Director and Publisher: Jack Artenstein
Executive Editor: Peter Hoffman
Director of Publishing Services: Rena Copperman
Managing Editor: Jama Carter
Editor: Claudia McCowan
Project Editor: Judith Liggett
Text Design by Wendy Staroba Loreen

Printed in the United States of America

International Standard Book Number: 0-658-00701-7

   01 02 03 04 DHD 18 17 16 15 14 13 12 11 10 9 8 7 6 5 4 3 2

Contents

Introduction

Irritable bowel syndrome (IBS) is the name given to a general group of symptoms after more easily diagnosed bowel diseases have been eliminated through a series of tests. Some experts claim IBS is not a disease at all; others say it is psychosomatic, or "all in the head." Alternative treatments abound, including everything from positive thinking to herbs and acupuncture. Due to the irregularity of these symptoms, even the most questionable approaches have been credited as cures for IBS—that is, until the symptoms reemerge.

Because I am a biochemist and nutritionist, a book about IBS is something of a "natural" for me, concerning as it does the intestinal environment, which is influenced by food, exercise, emotions, drugs, and herbs, as well as our genetic makeup. Gender also plays a role. More women than men suffer from IBS; estimates range from two to one to as high as ten to one.

Like other diseases that strike women more often than men, such as various inflammatory diseases, IBS has been linked to high levels of stress and anxiety. What goes on in our heads—stress, anxiety, and emotions—influences our biochemistry, which in turn affects what goes on in our bowels.

You really don't ever cure an illness like IBS. Rather, through a long series of trials, you can learn how best to manage and relieve the condition so that it no longer takes a toll on the quality of your life.

WHAT IS IBS?

The symptoms physicians often lump into the category of functional gastrointestinal disorders are listed below. Every person will experience one or more of these symptoms at some time in her life. When any one (or several) of them appear regularly, a physician will diagnose a functional GI disorder.

Symptoms of Functional GI Disorders

- Abdominal pain
- Bloating
- Bowel incontinence
- Chest pain
- Constipation
- Diarrhea
- Gas
- Heartburn
- Mucusy stools
- Nausea
- Pain in anus
- Pain in rectum
- Pelvic pain
- Trouble swallowing
- Vomiting

IBS is the most common of the twenty-five functional GI disorders. IBS affects approximately 20 percent of all adults and about two women for every man. It apparently knows no ethnic or racial boundaries and has a worldwide distribution, although it's recognized more often in developed countries, probably because of greater access to medical care. It is usually reported and diagnosed after age twenty and before age thirty-five, most often by age thirty.

When your gastroenterologist tells you that you have IBS, it is a nice way of saying that he cannot tell you exactly what's wrong. In contrast, he can definitely tell you what *isn't* wrong. IBS is not Crohn's disease, nor is it diverticulosis or one of the several forms of colitis. It is possible to have IBS along with one or even two of those clearly diagnosable GI disorders; having IBS along with Crohn's disease is a very unpleasant circumstance. Some people diagnosed with mild Crohn's disease or colitis could really have IBS, however.

IBS is as if your bowels decided to become nonconformists and take on a life of their own—a life dedicated to giving you a hard time. Its symptoms include abdominal bloating, pain, and problems defecating, such as diarrhea and constipation. Alternating bouts of diarrhea and constipation are the most commonly reported symptom. Pain can be associated with bloating and diarrhea.

IBS is, by definition, a problem with the bowels. To gain control over this difficulty, it's helpful to understand the anatomy involved.

THE GASTROINTESTINAL (GI) TRACT

Think of the GI tract as a hollow tube surrounded by a body that supports all its functions. This marvelous tube starts at the mouth and continues to the anus. About 30 feet in length, it is responsible for processing all the food we eat so we can receive the nourishment required to sustain life. Residue from this process, called stools or feces, is eliminated through the anus. The entire process takes about one and a half to three days. This time frame varies, however; one approach to treating IBS is to increase the fiber in your diet, which should help you achieve the ideal twenty-four- to thirty-six-hour period.

The GI tract is anything but a simple pipe: it is one of the most complex systems in the body. It consists of five parts, each very important; trouble in just one can be trouble for the entire body. Figure I.1 shows a diagram of the GI tract.

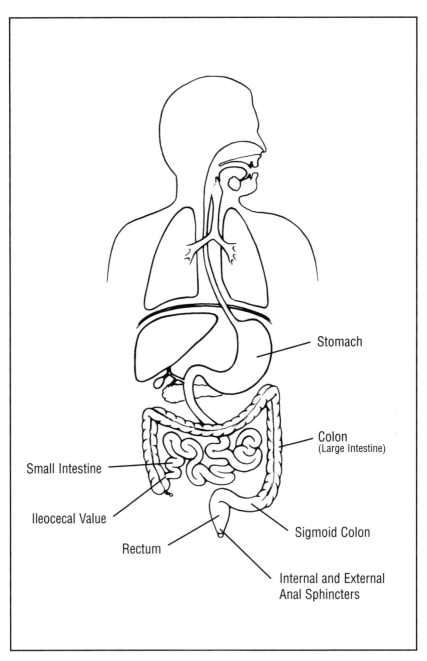

Stomach

Colon
(Large Intestine)

Small Intestine

Sigmoid Colon

Ileocecal Value

Rectum

Internal and External
Anal Sphincters

Figure I.1   **The GI Tract**

Illustration by Elizabeth Weadon Massari

Mouth and Pharynx

Digestion begins in the mouth. Chewing breaks ingested food into smaller parts so more surface area is exposed to digestive enzymes, catalysts that start the breakdown of starch, first in saliva and then in the stomach. Digestive enzymes are made and released (secreted) by the many glands found along the GI tract.

Esophagus

The esophagus is a tube about 1 foot long that connects the mouth to the stomach. By a muscle process called *peristalsis,* it moves the food from the mouth to the stomach. This wavelike motion pushes food along so well that you could eat a meal and complete digestion standing on your head.

Muscles surround the GI tract much like a rope wound around a hose. These muscles clamp down and in a synchronized, wavelike motion slowly move food along in each section of the digestive tract. If you want to get a feeling for how it works, get a piece of thin-walled rubber, cloth, or vinyl flexible tubing, and fill it with a soft but firm material such as bread or cookie dough, or soft clay. Wrap your fingers around it tightly and squeeze, moving the material along the tube. This is the same method a snake uses to move recently swallowed prey along its digestive tract; if you've ever watched a snake eat at the zoo or on a nature show, you should have a good idea of how the peristaltic process works.

When peristalsis becomes uncoordinated or hits a blockage, the muscles tense and pain follows. The pain is located in the abdomen as cramps. Cramps can vary from merely unpleasant to debilitating.

Stomach

Serious digestion begins in the stomach. More enzymes, secreted by the stomach lining, begin the breakdown of protein and fat. Food is acidified with hydrochloric acid, also released by the stomach lining, and kneaded by rhythmic motion into a mass (chyme) that will be passed on to the small intestine for complete digestion. The stomach contents become a grayish mass and are completely acidified by the time the stomach has finished its work.

Small Intestine

Through peristalsis, the stomach slowly passes its contents into the small intestine. The pancreas, a gland near the intestine, releases many enzymes that complete digestion. The gallbladder, located in the liver, releases bile acids into the small intestine via the bile duct. Bile acids act like detergents that allow the food materials, which consist of fat, protein, starches, and indigestible fiber, to mix thoroughly so enzymes can come in better contact with them. The enzymes break everything down to their smallest molecular parts.

The small intestine is about 20 feet long and is lined with myriad small, fingerlike, microscopic projections called *villi*. Villi make the actual surface area of the small intestine enormous and allow the completely digested nutrients from food to be absorbed. Along the lower one-third of the intestine water is also absorbed, so what leaves the small intestine is mostly undigested food material that is moist but not watery.

It takes about three to five hours for food to be digested and pass through the small intestine. Along with the food components, bile is reabsorbed and water is absorbed through the villi into blood vessels that transport them to the liver for further processing.

Large Intestine

If it takes food about five hours to go from the mouth through the small intestine, and about one to three days, on average, for undigested food material to be eliminated as stools, food must spend from one to two days—or even longer—in the large intestine.

The large intestine, or colon, consists of five distinct parts: the ascending colon, the large intestine junction, the transverse colon, the descending colon, and the rectum, which empties through the anus. IBS is primarily a disease of the large intestine.

Friendly bacteria, the intestinal flora, inhabit the large intestine and through a digestive process called *fermentation* break down some undigested plant starches and other materials. These microorganisms are essential because they produce about half the vitamin K we need. This is a perfect example of a symbiotic, or mutually beneficial, relationship; we get nutrition and they have a nice warm place to live. Technically, much of our feces consists of the cell walls of these intestinal microflora. (For information on these friendly bacteria and IBS relief, see chapter 24.)

Since little digestion takes place in the large intestine, one could ask, What is it good for? After all, there are people, such as cancer patients, some suffering from Crohn's disease, and accident victims, whose large intestines have been removed and replaced with small pouches they empty daily or with small openings on their sides, which empty into bags.

The answer is complex. When humans were much less technologically advanced, the nutrients derived from bacterial fermentation were probably much more important than today, when vitamin pills are available. Also, many anthropologists who study human origins and the survival of early humans believe that the ability to hold stools had tremendous survival value. Being able to hold stools until they could be deposited in a safe place (for example, into a stream) helped our early ancestors throw predators off the trail. The large intestine was and still is essential for water balance as well.

So the question is valid, but the answer is anything but simple. We are born with a large intestine and experience optimum vitality when it functions correctly. People who have to live without their large intestines can lead healthy lives, of course, but face inconvenient and sometimes uncomfortable alternatives.

GI Valves

When you mention a valve to a mechanic or engineer, he usually visualizes a mechanism that opens or closes an aperture. Heart valves, for instance, are actual flaps that cover or uncover openings in the heart so blood flows from one chamber to the other.

Valves in the digestive system are called *sphincters,* areas of muscle that can tighten or relax to allow contents to either flow or be held back. Visualize a place along the intestine, usually where one of the five sections connects to another, where there is a single large muscle that can clamp down and stop all flow completely, and you've got the picture. There are five sphincters:

1. *The upper esophageal sphincter* at the back of the mouth; this opens automatically when you swallow and allows food to move into the esophagus.

2. *The lower esophageal sphincter* at the base of the esophagus where it connects to the stomach; this opens during peristalsis to allow food to move from the esophagus into the stomach. This is a one-way valve that normally prevents the stomach contents from going the wrong way. As we all know, when we get sick, this sphincter doesn't always work properly.

3. *The pyloric sphincter* at the bottom of the stomach where it connects to the small intestine; this regulates the movement of the stomach contents into the small intestine.

4. *The ileocecal valve* where the small intestine enters the large intestine at the ascending colon; although a sphincter, it is called a valve and regulates the flow of materials entering the colon from the small intestine.

5. *Internal and external anal sphincters* at the base of the descending colon and anus; these two sphincters work together to allow passage of feces through the rectum and anus. These are the only two sphincters over which we have any control. They prevent unwanted defecation and allow us to control it.

SYMPTOMS OF IBS

The symptoms listed below are not consistent. In some people they are continuous, and in others they are intermittent.

Stools

In IBS, stools can be lumpy, so hard and dry that they're hard to move. They look like large rabbit stools and are called *scybalous stools*. They can also be loose and watery. Stools may be very narrow, almost like a long thin pencil. These stools result when the descending colon narrows during a spasm.

What that adds up to is sometimes straining to have a bowel movement and other times barely being able to get to the bathroom in time. Mucus often coats the stools or accompanies stools as a stringy mass, which can be enough to make you wonder if you have some strange disorder or even if your body is falling apart.

Problems with Bowel Movements

Bowel urgency may come at mealtime. Indeed, some IBS patients learn to eat only at home so they don't face the embarrassment of having to leave the table. The urge to move the bowels can strike at any time, however.

After a bowel movement, IBS sufferers often feel like there is more to be moved. This creates the problem of insecurity and straining, which is tough on the anus.

Bloating

Abdominal swelling is a real symptom of IBS, yet people with IBS don't produce more gas than average folks. They are simply more sensitive to any gas that is present; this could be due to weak musculature in the GI tract.

Abdominal Pain

Acute IBS attacks can cause severe abdominal pain. Pain often disappears with defecation. People with IBS often feel pain in the chest or throughout the entire abdomen. You can locate the source with a little effort, however. Doctors divide the abdomen into four sections. Draw imaginary horizontal and vertical lines on your abdomen using the belly button as the center where they cross. Let the four quadrants be the upper right, closest to your right arm, and lower right, closest to your right leg; the opposite for the upper and lower left quadrants.

A problem in the transverse colon, where it crosses the abdomen, is usually felt in the entire abdomen, although the two upper quadrants are often more tender. If you push on one of the lower quadrants, it will be felt in the upper quadrants as well, but not quite as intensely. Pain mostly in the lower left quadrant usually indicates a problem in the descending colon or around the rectum. Pain in the right quadrants is generally associated with a problem in the ascending colon. If you push on one of the other quadrants, you may feel pain there as well.

Pain and Bowel Movement

Does the pain follow or precede bowel function? For example, do you experience frequent, watery bowel movements and then pain? Or do you feel pain and then have a bowel movement that relieves it? Or perhaps you have a bowel movement that doesn't relieve the pain.

If the problem is located in the lower left quadrant, a bowel movement is more likely to relieve it simply because the descending colon can relax. In contrast, a bowel movement might not relieve a problem in the ascending or transverse colon.

If the colon clamps down tightly and stays that way in some area, it is called a *stricture*. A stricture is somewhat similar to a stiff or cramped muscle in your leg, except in the colon, it is squeezing down your colon to the size of a small tube in that area. It hurts just as a stiff or cramped leg muscle does.

When a stricture occurs in the descending colon, stools might appear long and thin. That is because the stricture has squeezed them down like the tube used by a pastry chef. When the buildup behind the stricture moves, the pain is likely to subside and the muscles can relax.

A stricture in another area, however, is not as likely to be relieved by a bowel movement. Those cases require time to relax and let the muscles return to their normal state.

Cramps

Since the peristaltic process is a continuous series of rhythmic, wave-like muscular contractions, when something goes wrong, the pain comes in waves. As the system tenses up or parts clamp down rather hard in some areas but is relaxed elsewhere, we get a cramp. Then, when it all relaxes again, the cramp subsides and we feel better. During a cramp it is not uncommon to sweat or for the forehead or face to feel wet and clammy; this illustrates how our minds and GI tracts are connected.

CAUSES OF IBS

If you've been diagnosed with IBS, obvious causes of GI distress, such as infection, an inflammatory disorder, blockage, or some other abnormality that can be detected by testing have been ruled out. That doesn't mean the symptoms aren't real; it simply means there are no *obvious* causes. Because IBS seems to have a family connection, family history is important (see chapter 1).

Anxiety and Stress

Stress is an integral factor in IBS. In fact, some experts claim the entire syndrome is nothing more than an exaggerated reaction to stress. This is a semipolite way of saying, "It's all in your head." Others say the stress results from the illness and produces ongoing tension, leading to a vicious spiral of stress, anxiety, and IBS symptoms.

It is difficult to say which comes first. Emotional upset probably triggers IBS attacks that, in their own way, cause stress, which leads to anxiety associated with the normal fear of real but vague symptoms. This fear and a lack of clear diagnosis is stressful by itself and increases the anxiety, which in turn makes the IBS worse. Breaking this vicious cycle will be explored in much more detail in later chapters of this book.

Gut Responders

Some people are known as "gut responders." For these people, emotional problems, stress, and anxiety bring on abdominal discomfort. The discomfort can range from minor cramping through outright nausea, bloating, severe cramps, diarrhea, and all the IBS symptoms.

This response varies from one IBS-afflicted individual to another as much as personalities vary in any group of people. Since about 70 percent of personality is hereditary, it follows that some GI responders have inherited that trait.

Foods

Some people find that certain foods will trigger an IBS flare-up. More commonly, however, an emotional upset or a very stressful event triggers the onset. Once started, some foods seem to make it worse. Basically, emotional upset initiates the episode, and certain foods exacerbate it. (For more on identifying and eliminating these "trigger" foods, see chapters 2 through 5.)

HOW TO USE THIS BOOK

If you find that one of the twenty-five ways to control IBS in this book helps you, don't automatically toss out the other practices.

Rather, consider each one carefully and, when appropriate, consider each as a way to improve your life. After all, IBS is not a precisely defined illness, and there is no single, exact approach that works for everyone.

Nevertheless, each idea described in this book can help. Together they can assist you to tame the tiger that hurts you. Each short chapter takes only a few minutes to read, and not a lot of effort is required to put the information into action.

The nutritional recommendations in this book should be followed by everyone, not only those with IBS, because good nutrition is the foundation of all health. By getting adequate fiber and sufficient vegetables, vitamins, minerals, and water, you eliminate one possible cause of IBS—poor nutrition.

Other chapters are similarly essential but should be approached with ongoing motivation. For example, dealing with stress is not something you can start, like taking a fiber supplement. Instead, you've got to analyze your situation, possibly keep a diary, and over time, come to the realization of how you cause internal stress and how your environment stresses you. It can be a very long process.

This book, while not an arduous read, contains all the ingredients you need to deal with your condition.

1

Establish a Genetic History

You and your doctor will understand your condition much better and be able to treat it more effectively once you establish whether you have a genetic, or family, history of a functional bowel disorder. If IBS has been a family trait in other generations, you and your doctor need that information. The more facts you have, the more likely you are to gain control over your condition. Prepare a good family history, listing your relatives who experienced this or a similar problem.

Because one in five adults has IBS to some degree, chances are good that there's a history of this condition lurking somewhere in your family tree. Indeed, modern epidemiological research on functional bowel disorders confirms this likelihood.

CONSTRUCT A FAMILY TREE

Draw a small circle (for example, trace around a penny) on the center of a piece of paper and write your name in the middle. Now, draw a circle about one inch larger around that and write in your parents' names and the names of your siblings. Draw another circle about an inch larger than the second circle and write in the names of your grandparents, uncles, and aunts. Finally, draw a circle about a half-inch larger and write in your cousins and great-grandparents (it doesn't matter, for this exercise, whether they are living). Your goal is to get information about each of these people. Ideally, you should speak to them personally, but if that is not possible, you can ask parents, sisters, brothers, close relatives, or friends. What you want to know is simple: Did they have a functional bowel disorder? Did they have persistent bowel problems?

Using the target you have just made as a guide, attempt to construct a family tree going as far back and as broadly as possible. Include both maternal and paternal sides of your family.

Try to interview as many of these relatives as you can. Explain that you've got a health problem; if you describe it well enough, they should "get the picture." Ask them the following pertinent questions about their bowel functions:

- Have they ever experienced:
  Constipation?
  Diarrhea?
  Alternating bouts of constipation and diarrhea?
  Occasional or frequent cramping?
  Mucus in stools?
- If so, at what age did onset occur?
- Did they ever go to an emergency room for abdominal pain?
- Were they ever diagnosed with a bowel disorder?
- Were they ever operated on for a bowel disorder, including appendicitis?

You will find that most people are quite helpful. Once you get going, expand the questions—as tactfully as possible—to include emotional issues:

- Did they ever have emotional disorders, such as depression and anxiety?

- Was medication ever required for emotional problems?
- Was there or is there alcohol abuse? (Alcoholics often suffer from diarrhea.)

IBS has emotional components; many experts classify it as a stress- and anxiety-related disorder. Therefore, it is important to find out if IBS or emotional difficulties occur in your family. It could be that some relatives have only one or the other. Some could be unlucky enough to have both.

If possible, you should also ask whether bowel or abdominal concerns ever interfered with their social or business lives. You are trying to find out if they ever encountered a situation that caused them to alter their interactions with other people. For example, would a salesperson avoid lunch or dinner meetings because she feared that either diarrhea or cramps would cause problems? Would a family member avoid invitations to dinner parties? Such habits may have become so automatic that they never classified the situation as a bowel disorder. When people alter their lifestyles to avoid these problems, they have a functional bowel disorder even if it's never been diagnosed. Lack of detection doesn't mean absence of an illness!

PUTTING IT ALL TOGETHER

Once you've gotten the information from all your relatives, map it out as follows:

- List your siblings and parents on one sheet of paper and note each one's response to these questions.
- List your mother's family on a separate paper and list your father's on another. You might learn that only one side of your family tree is burdened with bowel disorders. If you find that emotional problems occur on one side of the family and minor bowel disorders on the other, for instance, you

know you're an excellent candidate for all these difficulties to come together.

You might conclude, after all this research, that no one in your family except you has ever had this problem. Excellent! Take that information to your doctor because it is useful. It's unlikely, however, that you'll make such a discovery. Rather, you're likely to learn that you have a complex family history and that you're not alone in your situation.

2

Keep a Food Diary

Food selection is *your* responsibility. An enormous variety of food is available to you, so if you want to control your IBS you must consciously select food and food supplements that support rather than undermine good bowel health. The objective is to reduce diarrhea and constipation to an absolute minimum!

It is up to you to keep track of what, when, and why you eat, and to make positive adjustments that make you feel better. I can suggest foods and menus, but food choice at any given time is yours alone.

A food diary will put you in better touch with your body and its relationship to food than ever before. If you want to begin to control your IBS as quickly as possible, starting a food diary is the best way to jump right in.

Just as each journey—no matter how long—starts with the first step, each life accounts for an enormous amount of food, eaten one bite at a time. You are now going to make each bite work for you!

HOW THE DIARY WORKS

Once you begin keeping your diary and looking back over your entries, you'll probably discover that diarrhea or constipation is brought on by some foods and not by others. Obviously, you'll want to eliminate those foods that increase discomfort and increase those that don't. Then you will experience continued results, as food and food supplements make it easier for your body to get the nutrients that have the greatest benefit.

The advantage of keeping a food diary was vividly illustrated when a colleague at Georgetown Medical School and I conducted an experiment with students who wanted to lose weight. My colleague told his students I was doing some research on food habits and would like each of them to keep a food diary. Each was given a small diary in which he listed everything he ate and drank, as well as how much, when, and why. Then each night before retiring, each student was required to spend ten minutes reviewing what foods he'd eaten and to write a twenty-five-word summary critiquing his selections.

Every member of that group lost weight; two years later, all were slender, according to my colleague, who keeps in touch with them. They select food better than most dietitians. They enjoy all the food they eat and never go on diets. Each of them told me that the act of having to think through what he ate forced him to take control. Each recognized what he could do to control his eating habits and still relish food. These new habits now come to these individuals almost instinctively.

To start keeping your own food diary, purchase a small spiral notebook, preferably about 5 X 7, to fit into a pocket, purse, or briefcase. Record *what* you eat and drink, *how much, when,* and *why.* In addition, at the beginning of each day, note briefly how you feel—for example, constipated, bloated, crampy, and so on—and try to compare this with how you felt the previous morning. Do the same thing in the evening, but also evaluate your food in one or two sentences by answering: Was it good for you? Was it balanced? Did you eat enough? Did you eat too much?

There is no special format you need to follow. Just be sure to write what, when, why, and how you feel about your food—daily—no matter what you eat. And get in touch with how you feel.

I don't ask others to do things I don't test myself, so here is a sample entry from my own diary:

Date: May 13

Morning

What: One-half grapefruit, 6 ounces orange juice, oatmeal with zanta currants, 2 tablespoons flax oil, skim milk, two cups of tea with milk.

When: About 8:00 A.M.—I feel great.

Why: Feeling hungry after writing all morning—starting at 5:30 A.M. Broke at 7:00 A.M. to exercise.

What: Cup of tea, supplements (multiple vitamin-mineral, vitamin C, six omega-3 oil capsules, vitamin E), and an apple.

When: About 10:00 A.M.

Why: As a snack after a phone call from National Nutritional Education Society.

Afternoon

What: Tuna sandwich (with lemon juice, soy oil mayonnaise), apple, a cup of tea with milk.

When: About 12:30 P.M.

Why: Hungry. Just finished writing a chapter. Good time to break.

What: Tea with milk and an apple.

When: 3:45 P.M. with Jim—just talking.

Why: To take a break and pass the time pleasantly before my search for new winch for my boat.

Evening

What: Baked halibut steak (normal serving), salad, string beans, Italian bread, fruit pudding, tea as usual, and a Bosc pear.

When: About 7:30 P.M.

Why: Dinner with Nancy and Kim.

Critique: This was a good day. I feel fine. No aches, no pain.

I have seen people adopt many types of diaries; some have used commercial day planners, others have used elaborate computer recorders. Whatever works is fine. But remember the absolute essentials: honesty, keeping track of everything you eat, and paying attention to the results. And, of course, your end-of-the-day critique is the most important step of all. If done correctly, it will give you a better understanding of yourself and your relationship to food.

Since the update of my second book, *The New Arthritis Relief Diet,* was published, I've noticed that more physicians and diet experts have encouraged people to keep a food diary. This practice can really work for you in controlling your IBS, as well as in other aspects of your life.

One bonus from your food diary is that it will make you more conscious of the food you eat. You will learn more about what you put in your body and why.

People also tend to lose weight when they keep a food diary, if they were overweight to begin with. The reason is simple: People generally know what is good for them. Putting your eating habits in writing allows you to consciously start taking control of your diet.

3

Rule Out Lactose Intolerance

Anyone who has IBS should suspect lactose intolerance. That means the inability to digest lactose—the sugar found in mother's milk, cow's milk, and the milk of just about all other mammals. With a few exceptions, everyone is born with the ability to digest lactose. This ability changes as we age, however, challenging the notion that milk is a universal food good for everyone.

If you're lactose intolerant, you are unable to produce the enzyme lactase. This enzyme, normally produced by the pancreas when we're born, enters the small intestine and breaks milk sugar into the monosaccharides glucose and galactose, which are single sugars that can be absorbed from the small intestine into the blood. In the absence of lactase, lactose remains in the intestinal tract and upsets the normal water balance, which can cause diarrhea, abdominal cramps, bloating, and general abdominal upset.

Most Asians and Africans, and many Mediterranean people such as Greeks and Italians, start to lose the enzyme lactase at about age four; by the time they're teenagers the enzyme is usually gone completely. People of Northern European descent often lose the enzyme by age thirty-five or forty if they've stopped drinking milk; if they've continued to drink milk, the enzyme will usually stay with them.

People with functional bowel disorders, including IBS, are usually lactose intolerant. Lactose intolerance frequently accompanies chronic intestinal disorders, including Crohn's disease and colitis.

CHEESE AND YOGURT

In fermented dairy products, such as cheese and yogurt, most of the lactose is fermented and other sugars are produced; however, the protein and calcium of milk are still there. Most lactose-intolerant people can tolerate a few grams of lactose, which means they can use milk in coffee and tea and even drink a small glassful with no side effects, so the small amount of remaining lactose found in cheese and yogurt is not a problem. Cheese is a little high in calories and fat, however, so it should be used in moderation. Yogurt is an excellent alternative. Some people use yogurt in place of milk on cereal.

Certain people, however, seem to have a supersensitivity to lactose (or possibly to other factors in milk) and can't tolerate dairy products at all. These people should simply avoid dairy products altogether, or at least experiment with taking a lactase enzyme.

LACTASE PRODUCTS

Why not simply add the enzyme lactase to milk and break down the lactose to glucose and galactose? That's exactly what some people do. If you're lactose intolerant, you have three alternatives, all sold under the brand name Lactaid.

Lactaid brand milk is treated at the dairy with the enzyme lactase, which breaks the lactose down into glucose and galactose. It is sold in most supermarkets. More than 70 percent of the lactose has been eliminated; the remaining 30 percent should not be a problem. Eight ounces of milk contain about 6 grams of lactose. If 70 percent is broken into glucose and galactose, only 1.8 grams of lactose remain—not enough to cause a reaction in most lactose-intolerant people. If the remaining 30 percent of lactose is a problem, however, it can be totally eliminated by adding Lactaid lactase drops.

Lactaid drops is a liquid preparation of the enzyme lactase. When added to milk, these drops eliminate more than 99 percent of the lactose. So, if you're lactose intolerant and use Lactaid drops according to the directions, you can drink milk! There will be no symptoms of lactose intolerance, and you'll get all the nutrition that milk can provide.

The third option, *Lactaid caplets,* is a preparation of the enzyme lactase and is designed to work in the human stomach and small intestine. You simply take from one-half to three caplets at the beginning of a meal, depending on the amount of milk you intend to drink.

OTHER ALTERNATIVES

Every supermarket carries several alternatives to cow's milk. These beverages are usually called soy beverage or soy milk, rice milk, or almond milk. They are also offered in low-fat and reduced-fat choices. They are excellent milk alternatives and have many nutritionally desirable features.

Soy beverage is an outstanding milk substitute on cereals and delivers an extra bonus. Soy has many substances that reduce cancer risk and has been proven to contribute to the low rate of breast, prostate, and other cancers found in Asian countries.

SUGAR ALCOHOL INTOLERANCE

Sugar alcohols, including xylitol, sorbitol, and maltitol, are sweet alcohols that occur in small quantities naturally in most fruits; these small quantities are easily metabolized by our bodies. In many people, however, they cause discomfort when taken in larger amounts.

Sugar alcohols, especially sorbitol and maltitol, are used in some confection products and liquid vitamin preparations. There's no product similar to Lactaid for sugar alcohol intolerance. Therefore, read ingredients lists. If sorbitol, maltitol, or xylitol appears on the ingredients list of a product, use it cautiously.

4

Identify Food Triggers

Keeping a food diary for a month (see chapter 2) should tell you a great deal about yourself and your illness. Examining why you ate a particular food and when teaches you a lot about your habits. It can tell you the degree to which you do or do not live by the clock. Most important, it can help you identify foods that can trigger a flare-up of IBS.

We discussed lactose, the common milk sugar that is a widely known food trigger, in chapter 3. There are other foods and food components, in addition, that can cause a response to varying degrees. These "caution" foods are for your personal experimentation; some people can handle them and others will experience a negative effect, such as a flare-up. Most of these foods are carbohydrates.

SIMPLE CARBOHYDRATES

Carbohydrates generally fall into three groups: monosaccharides, disaccharides, and polysaccharides, or starches. *Mono* means "one," so monosaccharides consist of one unit, usually glucose, fructose, or the galactose in milk sugar. In our bodies, monosaccharides are converted to glucose or directly metabolized to carbon dioxide and water for energy.

Disaccharides consist of two units and include lactose, which, as you know, is glucose and galactose; common table sugar; and sucrose, which consists of glucose and fructose. Sweetness usually derives from fructose (for example, table sugar is sweet because of its fructose content). Disaccharides are broken down into glucose and fructose in the intestine, and the fructose is metabolized for energy.

A small number of people are sensitive to fructose. Sweet fruits, such as pears, grapes, figs, dates, prunes, and plums, are rich in fructose. Fruit rarely triggers fructose sensitivity reactions, however, unless you seriously overindulge (for example, eating a lot of grapes or figs in one sitting). Many fruits contain sufficient fiber to balance their fructose levels.

Fructose is widely used in food processing as a sweetener. Seldom does it appear on ingredients labels as "fructose," however, because pure fructose is very expensive. It is more often listed as one of the following man-made additives: high fructose corn syrup, corn syrup, corn syrup solids, or corn sweeteners.

If you notice while looking back over your food diary that a large soft drink or fruit drink will send you to the toilet with acute diarrhea and cramps, it may very well be the corn sweetener used in the product.

Carbohydrate Malabsorption

If carbohydrates trigger your IBS symptoms, it does not mean that you have an allergy to carbohydrates. Rather, it signifies that you do not absorb certain carbohydrates, such as fructose, well. This is called *malabsorption.* By not absorbing sugars adequately while absorbing other food components, such as amino acids and fats, correctly, your intestinal fluid balance is upset. This fluid imbalance usually triggers diarrhea and the cramps that come with excessive peristaltic action. It can also lead to constipation, although this happens much more rarely.

Once you have established that you have a carbohydrate absorption problem, you can learn to eliminate foods that contain the carbohydrates that cause trouble. (We'll discuss an "elimination diet" in the next chapter.)

The Honey Test

If you suspect fructose is a problem sugar for you, perform this simple test with honey, which is almost pure fructose: Prepare a cup of tea, add 1 or 2 tablespoons of honey, and drink it down. If no flare-up of diarrhea occurs after a few hours, you can probably eliminate fructose as a trigger. You may want to perform the test again with double the amount of honey, just to be sure.

Common Table Sugar

Common table sugar, or sucrose, is a disaccharide that must be broken into glucose and fructose by sucrase, an enzyme your body makes. Rarely do people lack sufficient sucrase to break down sucrose, even when they've overindulged in sweets. For those few people, however, undigested sucrose can upset the body's water balance and cause diarrhea, much as lactose does. Even in those who can digest it, sucrose presents the intestinal flora with a feast, and their increased action can cause gas and diarrhea.

You can easily test your sensitivity to sucrose by lacing a bland meal with extra table sugar, as in the honey test above. If you are sensitive, you can probably continue to use table sugar in tea or coffee, but you should avoid sugary desserts.

WHEAT GLUTEN OR GLUTEN

If your food diary indicates that breakfast cereal, such as wheat bran or some other cereal such as oatmeal causes a flare-up, or that a pasta dinner sends you running, or that bread, even whole-wheat or rye bread, triggers your IBS, you could have a wheat gluten or simply a gluten sensitivity.

Suspect wheat gluten or gluten sensitivity if foods on the following list cause an IBS flare-up:

- Cereals with wheat, barley, or oats, but not corn
- Crackers made from wheat, barley, rye, or oats
- Breads (except cornbread)
- Pasta and noodles
- Flour (also whenever used as a thickening agent, as in creamed vegetables)
- Canned foods (beans, soups, and so on)
- Some processed meats (for example, bologna)
- Cakes, cookies, and many desserts
- Puddings
- Gravies

If your diary leads you to suspect that wheat gluten or gluten in general is your problem, try a corn cereal with soy beverage to eliminate lactose (corn doesn't contain gluten). Then, a day or so later, try a wheat cereal prepared the same way. If it causes a flare-up, try making oatmeal a couple days later. Try a little pasta after a few days and then some breads. Be sure to test these foods by themselves; for example, while testing cereals, eat only boiled or steamed vegetables and avoid bread and pasta.

Wheat gluten and gluten sensitivities can cause serious intestinal disturbances, and they require medical intervention. If you suspect a wheat or general gluten sensitivity, you absolutely must see a physician. Go to your doctor with your test results. List what you've done and the results you've experienced. Your doctor, especially a gastroenterologist, should be able to help. With more diagnosis, she will be able to direct you to a dietitian and other resources that can show you the way to a new life free of GI troubles.

BEANS

You may find that beans cause a flare-up. (Chances are in such a case that your symptoms are not necessarily diarrhea, but instead gas and cramps.) This reaction to beans is not usually caused by a simple carbohydrate, but a more complex type of starch called raffinose; some consider it a special type of fiber.

You can solve the problem in one of two ways. Products are available that will break these bean carbohydrates down and the problem will go away. The other approach is simply to avoid eating beans.

5

Go on an Elimination Diet

Keeping a food diary and testing yourself for lactose, wheat, and other possible food sensitivities are essential steps in relieving IBS. Another tool in your armamentarium against this condition is what is technically called an elimination diet. Do not confuse this with popularized weight-loss or general diets that go by the same name; a true elimination diet is a serious approach to identifying foods that aggravate IBS symptoms.

HOW AN ELIMINATION DIET WORKS

An elimination diet is really quite easy to follow. Start with a very bland diet; for instance, with "engineered" foods, such as liquid formulas like Ensure and some extra fiber, say, from Metamucil. Another approach is to start with the Janowitz Core Diet:

- One starch: rice or baked potato (only one!)
- One meat/protein: preferably chicken, baked, broiled, or poached. Alternatively, select lamb, either broiled or baked.

- One canned fruit: Bartlett pears are recommended; peaches should also work.
- Use bottled mineral water if your tap water isn't of good quality.

Then carefully add potential trigger foods back into your diet, one at a time. Food sensitivities vary widely. For example, a person with egg sensitivity might be able to eat one egg a day, but when that person eats two or possibly three eggs in a row, she'll have a flare-up. Alternatively, if she eats two eggs in one sitting, she might have an immediate flare-up. This dictates the need for careful patience in following an elimination diet.

In contrast to food sensitivity, a food allergy produces an immediate, often devastating, reaction. An IBS flare-up is more likely to be due to a food sensitivity than to a food allergy, and identifying foods that cause flare-ups requires more time, up to several days. A good rule is to stick with a dietary intervention (for example, to keep suspect foods out of your diet) for at least three consecutive days, assuming you don't have a flare-up during that time, and note anything that happens on the fourth day. To be thorough, keep up the intervention for a full week. If there is no problem in a week, you can be sure the food at issue is safe.

When reintroducing real foods, be sure to look at entire food groups, such as vegetables, fruits, grains, and so forth. It is generally best to use natural, unprocessed foods. Vegetables should be cooked and fruits should be ripe. If low-fat or nonfat versions of foods exist, as with milk, use those first to eliminate fat as a possible culprit. For cereals, brands such as All-Bran Buds or Fiber One are excellent sources of fiber; however, both are processed and therefore not good alternatives. Test oatmeal instead—the old-fashioned kind, not instant. For meats and protein, broil a hamburger or fish. Don't eat processed versions, such as sausages or breaded fish or chicken. Avoid frying.

If you are using the liquid diet as your base diet, skip that liquid meal whenever you add a food. For instance, if you decide to start the day with oatmeal and skim milk, skip the morning liquid breakfast. Don't add some other type of food that day.

Do not expect the elimination diet to be a painless experience. You will be reintroducing foods to your body that you haven't eaten in some time. You might have a little stomach rumbling or a feeling that something isn't quite right. Don't confuse these experiences with significant flare-ups—a bout of diarrhea, cramps, a genuine attack of IBS.

Chapter 16 outlines a very healthy, well-balanced diet. As you test various foods, try to develop a similar diet that causes no flare-ups or discomfort.

6

Reduce Your Caffeine Intake

Many people without IBS report that their second cup of coffee in the morning triggers a bowel movement. This is because caffeine, as a general central nervous system stimulant, stimulates peristaltic motion. One cup of coffee delivers about 100 to 150 milligrams of caffeine; two cups of coffee supply 200 to 300 milligrams of caffeine, which, in a short period of time, is more than enough to stimulate peristaltic motion in an average person who weighs under 180 pounds.

A person with IBS may be no more sensitive to caffeine than the average individual; however, the sudden rush of caffeine "kick-starts" peristaltic motion and can cause IBS to flare up. The flare-up may be no more than a passing bout of heavy-duty diarrhea. If the rapid peristaltic motion meets some stubborn stool, cramps can result. There is one way to stop this cycle if you find this happens to you: reduce your caffeine intake.

TEST CAFFEINE

If from experience you suspect that caffeine or coffee or both triggers your IBS, test your hypothesis. You'll do this by testing various caffeinated beverages on separate mornings.

Always have two cups of the beverage indicated within thirty minutes, with plain toast. Don't eat for one hour following.

Day One: Brew 2 cups of coffee (1 tablespoon of ground coffee for each cup). If IBS is triggered, continue to Day Two.

Day Two: Brew 2 cups of decaffeinated coffee. If no IBS is triggered in one hour, drink 2 cups of regular coffee. If IBS is triggered, continue to Day Three.

Day Three: 2 cups of hot tea, steeped for five minutes. If no IBS is triggered in one hour, drink 2 more cups. If no IBS is triggered in the hour following, drink an additional 2 cups. If no IBS is triggered on the third day, go on to Day Four.

Day Four: 4 cups of hot tea, steeped for five minutes. If no IBS is triggered, stop.

If you react to regular brewed coffee but not to decaffeinated, you can rule out some other component of coffee as the culprit behind your flare-ups. Modern decaffeinated coffee is made from regular coffee beans with only the caffeine removed by steam extraction, so most of the oils and other materials remain. In some people, these other materials, especially the coffee oils, cause GI difficulty. If you respond to decaffeinated as you respond to regular coffee, then you are sensitive to something else in the coffee. Avoid all coffee, caffeinated or not.

Tea provides about 35 to 50 milligrams of caffeine, so two cups might not trigger IBS. If drinking four cups within thirty minutes doesn't trigger IBS, however, then you have established that the milder substances in tea provide a buffer for your GI tract; indeed, you have also established tea as an alternative stimulant beverage for yourself that can be used without a flare-up. Tea contains an ingredient called tannin, which has a mild astringent effect and could quite possibly modulate the caffeine effect. In clinical research, tea tannins have been able to reduce the gastrointestinal effects of some irritants.

CAFFEINE AND THE NERVOUS SYSTEM

Caffeine is a general central nervous system stimulant that activates alertness in average people. Some people are much more sensitive to caffeine than others, and for them a cup of coffee can trigger the "jitters" or some clearly increased nervous system activity.

Since experts recognize that a person's mental state affects IBS, caffeine's ability to stimulate the central nervous system could be a factor. If this is the case, symptoms won't show up following a cup or two of coffee, however. Instead, this might require the third or fourth cup, or might occur only when you've had a cup of coffee late in the day.

It takes your body about three hours to metabolize about half the caffeine in one cup of coffee. This means that drinking a cup of coffee every few hours, as people often do in the workplace and socially, slowly builds the level of caffeine in the blood. If no caffeine is taken after about four in the afternoon, its level is reduced to about one-fourth by 10:00 P.M.; if you use coffee or other caffeinated beverages in moderation, this should be a relatively minor amount. By the time you're into deep sleep (the REM stage), there is not enough caffeine in your system to significantly affect you.

If you're sensitive to caffeine, however, and your liver can't metabolize it away quite as rapidly as that of the average person, it will interfere with your deep sleep. The anxiety produced by poor sleep could in turn increase your general stress level and trigger an IBS flare-up.

Evaluating whether this subtle caffeine/stress cycle is contributing to your IBS can be very difficult. It is better to rule it out altogether by limiting your caffeine intake.

TEA AND SOFT DRINKS

A cup of standard black tea, made by steeping a tea bag or a teaspoonful of loose tea for about five minutes, provides 35 to 50 milligrams of caffeine per cup and is enough to provide the morning pickup for which many turn to coffee. Two cups of strong tea will provide the equivalent of only one cup of coffee. By drinking tea instead of coffee, you automatically limit your amount of caffeine because you can only drink so much fluid.

Many soft drinks provide about 35 milligrams of caffeine per 8 ounces. So, you could easily drink two cans of a soft drink in the morning and be drinking the equivalent of only one-half to three-quarters of a cup of coffee.

CAFFEINE ADDICTION

If you find that simply cutting back on caffeine is too difficult, you may be addicted, regardless of whether you drink coffee, tea, or soft drinks. Caffeine addicts who quit experience all the symptoms of narcotic drug withdrawal (albeit quite a lot milder), including anxiety, jitters, headaches, irritability, and general misery.

Caffeine withdrawal requires about a week—two at the most. If you find that you are addicted, you may want to strongly consider giving up caffeine entirely.

Caffeine in and of itself is not bad; in fact, it has been used as a stimulant for about 10,000 years. It definitely provides a nice pickup and stimulates alertness. Excessive use can cause nervous problems as well as addiction and will definitely aggravate IBS, however. The best course, particularly for those with IBS, is to consume caffeine only in moderation.

7

Eliminate Excess Alcohol

Alcohol has many effects on the body. When taken in moderation, alcohol, particularly wine, may help reduce heart disease risk. When taken in excess, however, it can cause diarrhea in people with bowel disorders as well as those without. It also has another, more insidious effect—it increases the amount of emotional and physical stress you experience. Stress is a major factor in IBS, so anything that increases stress should be avoided.

Alcohol is a toxin because it crosses the blood-brain barrier and at high enough levels can cause the brain to stop functioning. Alcohol is absorbed directly from the stomach, so when a person drinks heavily, his blood alcohol level starts rising rapidly. If blood alcohol reaches a sufficiently high level, the person can pass out; if it continues to rise, the brain will shut down and the person will die.

When a person eats while drinking, blood alcohol doesn't rise as rapidly. (That is one good reason to drink socially because there tends to be food available at the same time.) You can't rely on food to prevent the effects of alcohol, however.

Because alcohol is a toxin, the body detoxifies it as quickly as possible by metabolizing (burning) it to carbon dioxide and water. In fact, when alcohol enters the blood, the liver stops metabolizing everything else and focuses on eliminating the alcohol. That means that any fat or carbohydrate circulating in the blood will have to wait until the alcohol is reduced to a manageable level. Excess blood fat is first stored in the liver; sugar simply stays in the blood, and its level continues to rise.

That is why regular excessive alcohol consumption causes fatty deposits in the liver, which leads to cirrhosis of the liver. The excess sugar is converted to fat and often winds up in the same place. In addition, the excessive sugar can cause a similar excess of insulin production, and when the alcohol is gone, the blood sugar drops. The drinker usually goes for more alcohol when this happens and a downward health spiral is set in motion.

Low blood sugar is one of the worst messages the brain can receive. It is a signal that the energy necessary to keep its critical processes going is dwindling. Anxiety follows that signal, which in no time manifests itself as irritability and erratic behavior. When blood sugar drops, the person usually eats more food or drinks more alcohol—neither of which is a good idea. This proves the old saying about alcohol: "Moderation is the only way to go!"

People who drink socially consume, on average, about 2 percent of their calories in alcoholic beverages, with no adverse effects. Active people who are physically fit can usually handle much more than 2 percent of calories from alcohol; probably 4 to 5 percent. If you're 5 feet 5 inches tall, you probably burn about 1,800 calories daily; if you're 6 feet tall, you use 2,200 calories or more daily. Two percent of these levels is 35 to 45 calories daily. One and a half ounces of whiskey contain 105 calories, and a 3½ ounce glass of wine has 75 calories of alcohol. What that translates to is a few drinks or glasses of wine or beer every week, probably on weekends or occasionally with dinner.

Since a healthy liver can process about 1 to 2 ounces of alcoholic beverages per hour, the social drinking described above is no problem. Indeed, in recent years scientists have found that one glass of wine daily or even a mixed drink or beer may reduce the risk of heart disease by helping to elevate a fraction of cholesterol designated as "good" cholesterol. Social drinking is not a bad habit and may actually have some health benefits.

HOW MUCH IS SAFE?

A woman about 5 foot 6 inches tall who weighs 120 to 130 pounds should be able to consume daily a glass or two of wine, or a mixed drink containing 1 ounce of whiskey, or a couple of beers. At a cocktail party, she should not exceed one alcoholic drink or glass of wine per hour. Larger people can drink proportionately more; for example, a 6-foot-3-inch-tall, 190-pound man can probably safely consume a third again as much. He could drink about 1½ drinks per hour.

Any dinner, office party, or cocktail party can easily provide a week's worth of calories from alcohol. Two glasses of wine at a holiday celebration is hardly excessive, but keep in mind that most adults exceed their legal limit to drive if they consume three drinks within one and a half hours.

Alcohol consumed excessively (over a drink per hour), particularly at lunch, can cause trouble during the remainder of the day. That is because it forces the body to set other caloric materials aside, namely sugar and fat, while it metabolizes the alcohol to carbon dioxide and water.

This type of drinking causes blood sugar shifts and encourages fatty deposits in the liver. A drop in blood sugar increases irritability, which usually sends the person so hampered to seek stimulants: more alcohol, tobacco, or even candy. Often a doctor, not fully understanding what is going on, will encourage a person claiming to feel down or irritable in the afternoon to suck on hard candy. Sucking on the candy keeps the blood sugar up, but it is simply hiding the difficulty, while speeding the emergence of Type 2 diabetes, liver problems, periodontal disease, and possibly high blood pressure as well.

Some people believe—erroneously—that taking extra B vitamins as supplements will speed the body's process of metabolizing alcohol because the B vitamins are critical to alcohol metabolism. This is not true! Drinking alcohol too rapidly makes the alcohol and its by-products build up in your body faster than they can be passed off; you'll feel lousy until they're gone, regardless of the amount of vitamin B in your system.

Exercise helps speed the elimination of alcohol from the body because it quickens metabolism. Alcohol makes it harder to exercise, however. Who goes to the gym after a three-martini lunch? One is much more likely to look for a couch and take a nap.

A hangover is usually the result of dehydration caused by excessive alcohol consumption and the elevated blood sugar that very often follows. Together, these often cause fitful sleep and a severe headache the following morning.

Some people claim that drinking water when they have a hangover makes them tipsy; it's really water intoxication that their dehydrated brains are experiencing as they return to a normal hydration level. Drinking one glass of water for every drink prevents most of these problems, but decreasing the booze is the best approach overall.

8

Avoid Capsicum and Senna

We're currently living in an herbal renaissance in which all things natural are automatically considered good by many people. Although many herbs and natural products can be helpful (chapter 15 lists herbs that can help your IBS by reducing stress, for example), many have serious, deleterious side effects. Two of these are capsicum and senna, both of which are used in many products, and both of which pose problems for people with IBS.

CAPSICUM

Capsicum can have two very serious effects on IBS: capsicum can stimulate the bowel, causing diarrhea and serious cramps, and it can be very irritating to the bowel tissues. Capsicum can literally burn these sensitive tissues. Its effects can be especially bad if there happens to be any break or raw spot in the intestinal tissue.

Some people believe that taking capsicum capsules will clear up ulcers and other GI disorders. This may work in some cases although it has never been tested. To apply that logic to IBS, however, could spell disaster. Stay away from these products!

SENNA

Senna is probably the most widely used herb today. Its active ingredients are strong laxatives that work by stimulating the bowel. Senna's active ingredients can also precipitate mucus secretion and cause fluid and minerals to be secreted into the large intestine. Consequently, incorrect use of senna during constipation can lead to diarrhea and cramps. It may also cause potassium loss. Caution is the watchword. Be sure to read the ingredients lists on laxative products to be certain they don't contain senna.

Senna Precautions

- Senna should not be used by pregnant women.
- Senna is inappropriate for children under the age of six.
- People with diarrhea, inflammatory bowel disease, or intestinal ulcers must not use senna.
- Senna should never be taken with other medications.

9

Lose Excess Weight

Excess weight characterizes affluent societies throughout the world, especially in the last decade. The United States is now the most affluent—and the most overweight—society that has ever existed. Over 50 percent of the U.S. population is overweight, and over half of these are seriously obese (20 percent above normal weight).

Excess weight increases and exacerbates all illnesses, especially those in which stress and anxiety are a component, such as IBS. Being overweight shortens life expectancy, increases heart disease and all associated risk factors, increases cancer risk, makes all illnesses worse, and slows recovery.

Stress is a major causative factor in being overweight, and at the same time excess weight places a stress on every system of the body, including the GI tract, making overweight people more prone to functional bowel disorders. Excess weight and stress become an insidious spiral from which only the most determined people can extract themselves, as illustrated in Figure 9.1.

Losing weight isn't easy. A poll taken just five years ago showed that over 70 percent of adults would like to lose about 10 pounds; in a more recent poll, 70 percent upped their desired weight loss to 12 to 15 pounds. Considering that over 50 percent of adults are

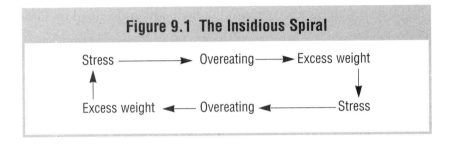

Figure 9.1 The Insidious Spiral

clinically overweight despite this desire, we can infer that losing weight is not an easy task. Even more difficult is keeping the weight off once it has been lost.

Often, people will say their excess weight is caused by some mysterious glandular disorder. That flies in the face of scientific evidence. Some studies have shown that some overweight people do have serious problems that cause them to eat excessively; however, 99 percent of overweight people can lose weight and keep it off once lost. Blaming our "glands" is not valid for all but a very small fraction of overweight people.

Losing weight and keeping it off has been proven over and over to improve health and longevity, as well as many chronic illnesses, such as high blood pressure, some functional bowel disorders, skin problems, and diabetes. We have much to gain by getting down to and maintaining a healthy weight.

THE ARITHMETIC OF EXCESS WEIGHT

A pound of body fat represents an accumulation of 3,500 excess calories; over some period of time, a person ate 3,500 more calories than she burned, and her efficient body stored those calories as fat for some future time when things might not be so good. When a person loses a pound, it means that over a period of time, she burned

3,500 more calories than she ate and her body simply used up some of those calories it had stored as fat for lean times.

Since most adults, when asked, say they would like to lose about 10 pounds, they have to create a 35,000-calorie deficit over some reasonable period of time, say, three to six weeks. (The time frame must be at least this long, because even very active people burn only about 3,000 calories daily. It's impossible to lose weight at a greater rate and still remain healthy.)

Creating a calorie deficit is just like creating a financial deficit; to do that, you simply spend more money than you take in. To create a calorie deficit, you simply have to burn more calories than you eat. It is that simple! No matter how many magical diets, magic pills, herbs, nostrums, and smooth-talking weight-loss gurus there are, weight loss comes down to a simple fact: Create a calorie deficit and you will lose weight.

Once you have lost weight, you won't gain it back—if you eat only as many calories as you burn.

CALORIES AND BASAL METABOLIC RATE

If you are overweight, it is because your body is overfat or conversely, your lean body mass (LBM), consisting of muscles, bones, and tissues, is too low for your weight. To lose weight, you need to lose fat and gain some more muscle.

Basal metabolism, the energy allocated to keeping the body functioning, burns the most calories during a twenty-four-hour day. For example, a 125-pound, reasonably active woman can get along well, neither gaining nor losing weight, on 1,800 calories each day. Of those 1,800 calories, about 1,200 go to basal metabolism. No matter what she is doing, even sleeping, her heart beats, her temperature remains normal, her kidneys remove wastes, her brain keeps everything working, she breathes, and all the myriad processes involved in living keep going, twenty-four hours a day. That's her basal metabolic rate (BMR).

Think of your automobile engine. Once started and left running, it will continually burn gasoline, even though it's sitting in one spot. The amount of gasoline burned depends on the engine size: a big eight-cylinder engine burns more than a four-cylinder engine. The higher your BMR (the bigger your engine), the more calories (fuel) you burn to keep running.

You can get a good picture of your BMR by consulting Table 9.1.

Burning Excess Calories

Physical activity, of course, burns calories in addition to your BMR.

- Sedentary activity (sitting) increases BMR by 0.2.
- Light activity increases BMR by 0.3.
- Heavy activity increases BMR by 0.4.

People recognize that regular exercise burns calories. Let's calculate how many calories exercise actually burns. Exercise burns calories in proportion to weight. Consider two levels of activity: a vigorous workout on an exercise machine that simulates cross-country skiing burns 0.03 to 0.04 calories per pound of body weight per minute; a moderate workout on a stair stepper burns 0.02 to 0.03 calories per pound of body weight per minute.

Now suppose two people, one a 130-pound woman and the other a 170-pound man, do each workout for thirty minutes apiece. In thirty minutes of vigorous exercise, the 130-pound woman burns about 137 calories (0.035 x 130 pounds x 30 minutes), while the 170-pound man burns about 179 calories (0.035 x 170 pounds x 30 minutes). In the thirty minutes of moderate exercise, the woman burns about 98 calories (0.025 x 130 pounds x 30 minutes), and the man burns about 128 (0.025 x 170 pounds x 30 minutes). Working hard and using lots of muscle groups can increase the amount of calories burned by 10 to 20 percent, but that still only

Table 9.1

Approximate Basal Metabolic Rate in Calories

Height	Weight*	Calories per 24 hours					
		Age 20	Age 30	Age 40	Age 50	Age 60	Age 70
FEMALE							
5 ft 2 in	110 lb	1234	1243	1211	1176	1137	1105
	130 lb	1339	1327	1293	1255	1213	1179
	150 lb	1423	1411	1375	1335	1290	1254
5 ft 5 in	125 lb	1372	1361	1326	1287	1244	1209
	145 lb	1457	1445	1408	1366	1321	1284
	165 lb	1542	1529	1489	1446	1398	1358
5 ft 7 in	135 lb	1457	1445	1400	1366	1321	1204
	155 lb	1542	1529	1489	1446	1398	1358
	175 lb	1627	1613	1571	1525	1475	1433
MALE							
5 ft 10 in	160 lb	1819	1715	1660	1632	1573	1491
	180 lb	1915	1805	1747	1718	1656	1570
	200 lb	2011	1895	1835	1804	1739	1648
6 ft	170 lb	1896	1787	1730	1701	1639	1554
	190 lb	1992	1877	1817	1787	1722	1632
	210 lb	2088	1967	1904	1873	1805	1711
6 ft 2 in	180 lb	1992	1877	1817	1787	1722	1632
	200 lb	2088	1967	1904	1873	1805	1711
	210 lb	2145	2021	1957	1925	1855	1758

* Three weights are given for each height: the first is ideal weight, the second is overweight, the third is obese. A formula for working out your ideal weight is as follows:

Females—multiply every inch over 5 feet by 5 and add 100.

Males—multiply every inch over 5 feet by 5 and add 110.

Note: Personal BMR varies from one person to another and can depend on heredity. It may also vary according to the environment: in cold weather the metabolic rate is higher to keep you warm; in warmer weather, depending on humidity, it has a tendency to be lower. The lower your body-fat percentage, the higher your metabolic rate will be.

increases the amount in our example to 164 calories for the woman and 215 calories for the man. As you can see, to burn off the 3,500 calories required to lose 1 pound of weight at these rates requires lots of willpower and self-discipline.

The real way that exercise contributes to weight loss is by converting fat to muscle. Muscle has a high BMR because it's active tissue; fat, which is storage tissue, has no BMR. If you exercise and diet together, you will find the weight comes off faster; in addition, you don't have to lose as much because muscle looks nicer than fat. Not only will exercise improve IBS and speed weight loss, it also improves general health.

Some additional energy gets used simply digesting your food. For example, you don't gain any calories by eating celery; in fact, you lose some. (You also lose more calories to digestion if you are emotionally upset.) Most experts estimate this loss at about 10 percent of BMR.

The two practical examples in Table 9.2 will give you a good idea of the energy expenditure during a typical day for two people: a 170-pound man and a 130-pound woman.

DIETING DOES WORK

Just about every day, a new diet comes on the market that purports to work better than every other diet. Logic tells you that if these diets worked—and most do, to some extent—there must be something about losing and keeping weight off that goes beyond caloric balance.

Weight is always a complex interaction of heredity and environmental factors so subtle as to defy complete analysis. Superimposed on all that complexity is how society uses food: for pleasure, conducting business, social interaction, and even family fellowship. In addition, advertising hits us from every direction and about 95 per-

Table 9.2

Daily Energy in Two Lives

	170-pound man	130-pound woman
BMR	1787	1327
Work energy: Light (salesperson/teacher)	536	398
Energy lost to food	179	133
Exercise: Vigorous for 30 minutes	153	117
Total energy in calories	2655	1975

cent of food advertising is for foods that deliver lots of calories with little nutritional value.

So, the problem with dieting is that once you've lost the weight, you must return to the world that caused you to gain weight in the first place. That is why dieters usually gain back what they've lost, plus a little extra.

Worse is the rate at which weight loss can be sustained. If a person follows a typical fad diet, say, the latest high-protein diet, he will lose a lot of weight, up to 5 percent of body weight, in the first week. After that it comes off at about 1.5 to 2.5 pounds per week, depending on how overweight he was to begin with.

Therefore, losing 50 pounds, which were probably put on over a few years, takes at least fifteen to twenty weeks, or about five months. Dieting for that long takes willpower that will challenge even the most dedicated dieter.

Don't get pessimistic, however, because there is a plan that works. It is so deceptively simple that few people use it, but those who do always succeed.

Food Diary and Fat Bags

In chapter 2, we discussed food diaries. In addition to helping you pinpoint the patterns and causes of your IBS, your food diary can be a valuable tool in weight loss.

Whether you keep it for IBS control or weight loss, the food diary must include everything you eat, as well as why you eat it, when you eat it, and any special circumstances. Pretty soon you'll start understanding why you eat what you do. Use the critique each day to help you see where you can do better and where to apply willpower.

In addition, keep track of the daily weather and temperatures. On cold or rainy days, people tend to eat more. Becoming aware of this pattern will allow you to find alternative outlets.

Fat bags are another simple device that helped people lose weight in the medical study mentioned in chapter 2. Each person was instructed to purchase a pound of sand for each pound he wanted to lose, as well as a cloth bag, called a fat bag. For each pound that came off, a pound of sand was put in the fat bag, which was displayed prominently. Some people displayed their fat bags at work, much like people keep family photos on their desks. The fat bag is essentially a trophy you can give yourself and show others.

It also pays to join or organize a weight-loss group whose members have to "weigh in" each week. The motivation of the round of applause you get for each lost pound, added to the fat bag trophy, is enough to boost anyone's willpower.

The bottom line is simple. Gain control of your emotions and eat sensibly so you will lose the weight you must and keep it off permanently.

10

Exercise

Regular exercise provides two major benefits for IBS sufferers, so important that neither can be overemphasized:

1. Exercise dramatically improves regularity.
2. Exercise reduces the emotional stress that can lead to IBS flare-ups.

REGULARITY

Correct exercise improves cardiovascular tone; that is, it improves the heart and the circulatory and respiratory systems. Regular exercise also improves and tones all the muscles in the body, including the GI muscles.

People who exercise routinely usually notice that their bowels move regularly. Those who exercise in the morning usually report their bowels move before, or soon after, they exercise. People who exercise late in the day, generally after work, similarly report better bowel regularity and that the movement occurs most often in the mornings. Exercise physiologists have studied and confirmed this regularity.

EMOTIONAL EFFECTS

Some experts claim that IBS is at least 50 percent emotional. Stress, they say, results from a combination of anxiety, inability to handle life's complexities, and a lack of free time to simply wind down. Exercise is essential in reducing the effects of stress. People who exercise regularly handle stress more effectively and are much less likely to become anxious than those who don't.

AEROBIC VERSUS ANAEROBIC EXERCISE

Aerobic means "with air"; *anaerobic* means "without air." "Anaerobic exercise" is a slight misnomer; you breathe when you do anaerobic exercise just as when you do aerobic exercise, but you don't exercise your heart and arteries as much as elevate your general metabolism.

Anaerobic exercise is usually short in duration, even if it is quite vigorous. Your body performs almost without the need for you to breathe. For example, running a 100-yard dash is vigorous and leaves the runner gulping for air; it is anaerobic because the energy comes from the metabolism of energy-yielding materials within the body rather than from inhaled oxygen.

Weight lifting is another typical example of anaerobic exercise. Everyone experiences anaerobic exercise when they run up a flight of stairs or to catch a bus.

In contrast, aerobic exercise is done for longer periods, and energy is dependent on the air breathed during the exercise. Walking briskly for forty to sixty minutes, jogging for fifteen or more minutes, or swimming are all examples of aerobic exercise that require regular breathing and, when finished, might not leave the person out of breath even if he is sweating profusely.

By elevating general metabolism in aerobic exercise, you build your cardiovascular system. Your heart and arteries—indeed, your entire cardiovascular system—are mostly muscle and require exercise more than any other system in your body. By doing some form of aerobic exercise, you prevent the buildup of fatty deposits and may even remove some. These deposits are the foundations of heart disease; preventing or eliminating them through exercise is one of the most important ways you can prevent this disorder. Exercise also prevents high blood pressure, Type 2 diabetes, and other illnesses.

Anaerobic exercise works large muscle groups, such as the arms and legs, challenging the cardiovascular system. In this way, major muscle groups and the cardiovascular system are conditioned together. Aerobic fitness produces entire body fitness. In contrast, a weight lifter can strengthen one muscle group, but might not condition his cardiovascular system unless he also does aerobic exercise.

TRAINING EFFECT

Training effect is scientific jargon for what results when you have exercised and improved your cardiovascular system, as you do in aerobic exercise. You probably also have helped to build muscles, such as those in your legs and arms, in the process. When you finish, you are in better condition than when you started. Seems worth doing, doesn't it?

To get a training effect, you must:

- Achieve a training heart rate quickly and do the exercise for at least twelve minutes and preferably twenty minutes, or
- Achieve an increased heart rate and keep it up for at least thirty minutes and preferably one hour, or
- Combine the above two requirements by achieving a modest increased heart rate and keeping it up for at least twenty minutes and preferably forty minutes.

Exercise is effective only when it is done regularly and with some rest periods, such as a day off every three or four days. You should exercise on five out of every seven days. Once you have been

Table 10.1

Training Heart Rates for Average People

Age	Maximum	75% Maximum	10-second Pulse
20	200	150	25
25	195	146	24
30	190	143	24
35	186	140	23
40	182	140	23
45	179	134	22
50	175	131	22
55	171	128	21
60	160	120	20
Over 65	150	113	19

exercising one way regularly for a year and are in good shape, it is an excellent idea to use a variety of forms of aerobic exercise on different days, or weeks, to increase fitness. You will improve because each type of exercise has its own benefits.

While exercising, the temperature inside your muscles increases to about 102 degrees from its normal 98.6 degrees Fahrenheit. That 3.4-degree rise (1 percent) raises the rate of metabolism over 17 percent, which increases circulation by at least 100 percent. This change in circulation brings more oxygen to all organs and tissues, including the brain, and, at the same time, flushes wastes (toxins) from your body. It is like a spring rain cleaning dirty streets; this is why regular exercise reduces the risk of just about every known disease.

A training heart rate is about 70 to 80 percent of the maximum rate your heart can beat safely. If you want to be precise in your exercise you should achieve this rate and keep it up for about twenty to thirty minutes. Table 10.1 shows the training heart rates for average people.

Suppose you can't jog or don't have access to a pool or stair stepper or for some other reason can't exercise vigorously enough to achieve a training heart rate. No problem: a brisk forty- to sixty-minute walk will impart a training effect, even though the heart rate is below the training level. Some people can't get to a training rate easily. Some also need to exercise longer in each session. If you're one of these people, you must work a little harder to keep the gift of health you have and do even more work to make it better. Although working harder can mean running or walking faster, doing it longer is better; then you don't place as much wear and tear on your joints.

WHICH AEROBIC EXERCISE IS BEST?

Most people can take a brisk hike, jog, cycle, or swim. Nowadays there are devices that simulate just about every type of exercise and can be used at home or in gyms. Table 10.2 lists the best types of aerobic exercise and the approximate time required for a significant training effect.

Table 10.2

Time Required for Exercise

Exercise	Time Required
Brisk walk	12 minutes per mile for 40 to 50 minutes
Jogging	8 minutes per mile for 25 minutes
Bicycling	25 minutes at 13 mph
NordicTrack or actual cross-country skiing	25 minutes
A leg-and-arm rowing machine or actually rowing in a boat with a movable seat	25 minutes
Aerobic Rider	30 minutes
Swimming laps with regular strokes	30 minutes or 50 minutes if you are slow
Stair stepper	30 minutes

WHAT TIME OF DAY IS BEST?

The best time of day to exercise is open to debate: physiology gives the edge to the end of the day and sociology to the beginning of the day.

Exercise not only tones the body, it relieves stress and tones the mind. Stress for most people is usually highest at the end of the day, so exercise then helps the mind as much as the muscles.

Early-morning exercise, however, provides a different advantage. Any time you exercise, your brain produces natural opiates called endorphins that elevate your mood so you become more optimistic. Although they help you feel better after the day is done, they also help you start the day with an optimistic outlook. So, even if evening is biologically a little better for exercise to relieve stress and eliminate toxins, its edge isn't large.

Sociologists have learned that people who exercise in the morning are less likely to quit, because most people have control of the early morning hours before the day's obligations take over. All you have to do is rise earlier and get started. Most studies also have shown that morning exercise makes you more efficient during the day. Whatever time of day you choose, the important thing is to exercise.

START NOW

By the time you finish reading this paragraph, you will have 100,000 new blood cells and about 14,000,000 other new cells. They can use the extra air to function efficiently. If you haven't been exercising, start slowly; a brisk forty-minute walk is an excellent way to begin. Then progress to brisk walking for five minutes, then a one-minute jog followed by five minutes walking, and continue in this manner for up to forty minutes. A healthy person with no leg or heart problems can maintain a twelve-to-fifteen-minutes-per-mile pace for forty minutes, or about 2.5 or 3.0 miles. A practiced, brisk walker will do ten minutes per mile. You can follow the same pattern with a stationary bicycle or any other device.

11

Explore the Mind-Gut Connection

As any IBS sufferer can tell you, IBS symptoms are real! Some symptoms and flare-ups, however, originate in or are worsened by your emotions, level of stress, or anxiety. We all know people who get sick at the sight of blood or during a bumpy airplane flight; these situations prove there is a connection between our psychic activity and what goes on in our guts.

SOMATOFORM DISORDERS

A *somatoform disorder* has persistent symptoms severe enough to interfere with day-to-day living and cause visits to the doctor, but which cannot be definitely attributed to a particular medical condition. Symptoms of somatoform disorders include:

- Digestive problems
- Fatigue
- Insomnia
- Headaches
- Fainting or almost fainting

- Dizziness
- Heartbeat problems (racing, pounding, fluttering)
- Pain in back or chest, or menstrual pain
- Sexual dysfunction (painful intercourse for women; impotence for men)
- Unresolved pain in an extremity or shoulder

We all have one or more or all of these symptoms at one time or another, but they usually pass. If one persists, we go to the doctor. If the doctor cannot diagnose a specific illness or other cause, he concludes that it is a somatoform disorder. Irritable bowel syndrome is such a diagnosis.

To understand the relationship between your IBS and your emotions, you must be very honest with yourself and ask yourself some very blunt questions.

ALCOHOL

Do you allow alcohol to control some aspects of your life? Here are some questions you should consider:

- Do I need a drink at a certain time every day or on certain days?
- Do I drink excessively under certain conditions; for example, in groups or around certain people?
- Do I drink alone regularly?
- Do I sometimes need a drink to get started?
- Do I ever receive criticism about my drinking or has someone told me to cut down?
- Do I ever feel guilty about drinking or resolve to cut back on my alcohol intake?

A "yes" to several of the above questions should be your cue to get help for alcohol abuse. Solving that problem may very well resolve your IBS completely. Alcohol and IBS have a physiological connection; excessive alcohol can precipitate a flare-up of diarrhea. In addition, if alcohol is an essential part of your life, there may be some emotional upset that you are covering up with alcohol. Dealing with that upset in a constructive way may eradicate a root cause of your IBS.

DEPRESSION

Being human means that there are times in life when you'll feel depressed. After all, things don't go right all the time: sometimes we lose; sometimes we lose a person who's close to us; sometimes things don't work out the way we hoped they would. Bad things do happen to good people; that's life. We get through those periods, recover, and go on with life. This is situational depression, which everyone faces from time to time. Clinical depression, on the other hand, seemingly comes from nowhere and interferes with our lives.

Many tests exist to detect depression, and mental health professionals will use one or more of these tests to uncover depression in their patients. If you think you may be suffering from depression, answer the following questions honestly:

- Do you feel down when others around you are normal or even up?
- Do you feel sad even if you haven't experienced any loss or received any bad news?
- Does everything you do seem like work? Do you lack interest or enthusiasm, or is there little or no pleasure in daily activities?
- Do you experience periods during which you have trouble falling asleep or staying asleep? Conversely, once asleep, can you sleep beyond a good night's rest? If not awakened by an alarm or someone else, would you simply remain asleep?

- Do you feel fatigued even when you've had ample rest?
  Or, is your energy level low?
- Do you fidget or are you restless? Do you find it hard to
  listen attentively?
- Do you believe you are failing, not achieving, or that you
  haven't measured up to your potential, or to other's
  expectations? Do these feelings elicit guilt?
- Do you concentrate on the task or objective at hand? Do you
  find it difficult to think about issues or problems? Do
  decisions come hard?
- Do you contemplate suicide when things are normal? For
  example, if your spouse just asked for a divorce, you might
  momentarily consider suicide; don't include such situations
  in your answer to this question. Rather, do you ever think
  about suicide when there is no clear reason for it?

If you answer yes to any four of these questions, especially the
first two, then you may be depressed. You should discuss this with
your doctor and request a referral to a professional who can correctly
diagnose and treat your condition.

ANXIETY

Anxiety often develops from excessive stress. It can also be a component of a complex disorder that develops in part because you have
a physical illness that seems unresolved—your IBS. Anxiety affects
everyone from time to time. If the symptoms persist or have almost
become a general part of your personality, however, you could be
suffering from chronic anxiety. Answer the following questions:

- Have you felt your environment has been out of control regularly for several months? This relates to those things you do
  have some control over, such as family, work, home, and so on.

- Are you irritable a large percentage of the time? Can you greet people warmly and not snap at ordinary comments? Do you take kidding without feeling angry?
- Do you wake up tired? In short, does a reasonably good night's sleep restore your energy?
- Do you have trouble falling asleep? Staying asleep for most of the night?
- Are you always waiting for something that never seems to come or happen? Are you restless most of the time? Do your friends ask why you are on edge?
- Can you concentrate? If you have a task at hand, can you focus on it without difficulty and continue so as to move the task or project along?

If you answered yes to three of the above questions, you might be suffering from anxiety. As in depression, your doctor can direct you to a health care professional who can help you with the problem.

12

Identify and Neutralize Sources of Stress

Everyone lives with stress. Seemingly stress-free lives are dull, and boredom is itself a major stressor. We all therefore must learn to dissipate the effects stress has on our physical and mental health—particularly those of us living with IBS. It is important to identify our most common stress sources so we can neutralize their detrimental effects on our health.

INTERNAL SOURCES OF STRESS

Each person, consciously or unconsciously, creates his own internal stress. One individual may go through life unaware of political issues; another may lose sleep over every international situation. Others may live one step ahead of foreclosure yet remain unconcerned; the same people may become depressed if their children aren't very academically or athletically successful. A person might be so concerned about punctuality that he is always at least ten minutes early; another must be invited thirty minutes early to ensure he arrives on time.

You cannot change the world or the people that make it go around, but you can identify those things that cause you stress, eliminate or change those you can, and learn to live with those you can't.

Responses to Change

Change characterizes our society. A computer is considered out of date, if not obsolete, in less than three years. Similar attitudes are emerging about people. We are expected to take courses, to continue to learn new skills, or to hone our existing ones to maintain our value. Someone who doesn't change is said to be in a "rut." If you're considered one of those people, by yourself or by others, it can be stressful. We feel pressure to change, but at the same time various external demands conspire to keep us from doing so.

We tend to compartmentalize people, to classify them as knowing only one thing or as being effective in only one area, an attitude that is an indirect outcome of technology and increased specialization. Our world, which prizes change, often won't let people whose specialty is essential to the success and well-being of others evolve. If these people aren't content in their specialization, their lives can be continually stressful.

EXTERNAL SOURCES OF STRESS
Family

Family demographics are changing rapidly in our society; family members often have little or no control over many factors that affect family life, such as the availability of leisure time and the demands of work. The inability to control events that shape your life is stressful, for children as well as for adults.

If you're a parent, you can modify family behavior to reduce the stress in all your lives, often by simply setting basic rules and maintaining open communication.

Work

The greatest number of stressors most of us face is found in the work-place, which can include everything from the home, to the middle manager's office, to the bungee-jumping concession, to the airplane cockpit, to the sales desk.

Work stress varies for each individual. One homemaker might be upset when the children track dirt on the floor; another could hardly care less. One manager might work well under the cloud of a dead-line and is bored when objectives are poorly defined, and another might love to bring open-ended objectives to fruition quickly and work long hours just to do so.

Job stress also varies by occupation. In Table 12.1, I list various occupations from my study of stress-related illnesses, measured by their tendency to cause high blood pressure, cardiovascular disease, ulcers, and nervous disorders.

Table 12.1

Job Stress

More Stress-related Illnesses	Fewer Stress-related Illnesses
Laborer	Seamstress
Secretary	Checker
Lab technician	Craftsperson
Office manager	Maid (domestic)
Foreman	Farmhand
Manager	Equipment operator
Waiter	Child care worker
Machinist	Packer
Farm owner	Tenured university professor
Miner	Personnel worker
Painter	
Computer programmer	
Air traffic controller	

Table 12.1 suggests that the most stressful positions are those where performance is continuously appraised (secretary, laborer, lab technician, and so on); positions of responsibility in which your performance is dependent on others (manager, office manager, foreman); positions in which success is dependent on things outside of your control (farm owner); positions in which you are responsible for people's lives (air traffic controller).

Contrast these stressful situations with the less stressful jobs. Occupations in which a high level of expertise and self-confidence is required, often for tasks that can't be rushed (seamstress, craftsperson, equipment operator) are not as stressful; neither are positions in which you have a clear-cut job to do and no responsibility for failure (farmhand, packer); other positions that fall into this category are those with guaranteed job security and a great demand for expertise (tenured university professor), or with little competition (personnel worker, maid).

Ask yourself the following questions about your job:

• In the descriptions of stressful or less stressful jobs, where does your job fit?
• What can you do to make it less stressful?
• What aspects of your job must you simply learn to accept?

A working person's longevity is most clearly predicted by his work satisfaction, more so than by genetics, tobacco use, or any other measure. If longevity is affected by workplace dissatisfaction, it follows that illnesses are also affected. Somatoform illnesses such as IBS in particular may be aggravated.

Ways to handle unavoidable stressors, whether at work or at home, are discussed in the next few chapters.

13

Stop Internalizing Stress

People respond to stress in many ways; these can be broken down into two fundamental approaches: outwardly exploding and inwardly imploding.

Exploding, of course, is just an exaggerated way of describing dissipating stress through outwardly directed activity. For example, people who explode may speak their minds, go for a run or exercise, stand up and shout, beat the desk, and so on. In short, they find healthful ways to dissipate the mental and physiological by-products of stress that build up in their bodies.

People who implode, on the other hand, keep stress inside and don't find healthy ways to dissipate those stress by-products. Such people often show no outward reactions to situations, and others sometimes wonder if they have any emotions at all. Such people often develop GI tract problems as well. Are you one of them?

As we've learned, stress affects the GI tract. Crohn's disease is a good example of a stress-related GI disease; in a survey in which I asked one hundred Crohn's patients what caused a flare-up of their disease, 100 percent named stress as a causative factor. (Indeed, when filling out the questionnaire, some Crohn's patients wrote "STRESS" in large capital letters diagonally across the page to make the message impossible to miss.) Stress and IBS are similarly interrelated.

To determine if you've been internalizing stress and thereby increasing its detrimental effects on your IBS, ask yourself the following questions:

- Do I have a tendency to hold my anger inside in stressful situations?
- Do I keep my problems to myself?
- Do I harbor feelings of guilt?
- Do I feel I am going to be left out of things?
- Do I speak up when I am treated unfairly?

Look for patterns in your life in which you tend to implode rather than explode.

HEALTHY OUTLETS FOR STRESS

As we've learned, we are all subject to stress. How we deal with it determines much about our health. Consider the following healthy outlets for stress:

- Exercise. It's generally best to exercise at the end of the day, but any time of day is fine. Remember, some exercise is always better than none.
- Confronting stressors. Identify your sources of stress and find ways to neutralize them.
- Downtime. Allow yourself time to relax, think things through, and dissipate stress.
- Self-affirmation. Speak up for yourself and affirm your worth as an individual.

ASSERTIVENESS SEMINARS

If you find that you hold emotions inside, there are ways to change your behavior. Seek out a health professional who can both counsel you and direct you to assertiveness training where you can learn new responses to replace your current, imploding behavior. And don't be embarrassed to take such training if you need it! A golfer who's been slicing his drives will go to a pro to learn how to change his stroke; taking classes in assertiveness is really no different.

14

Avoid Marginalized Living

As life's complexities increase, the time people have for themselves diminishes. That is what health experts call *marginalized living*. Marginalizing means filling your life to the brim with tasks, plans, and deadlines, leaving no slack time to deal with crises or sudden problems or to spend on fun and hobbies. In too many cases, quality time with children, spouses, parents, and other family and friends is sacrificed.

Marginalized living is stressful living, and as we've learned, stressful living is closely linked to IBS. Learning to demarginalize your life can only relieve your IBS—and will probably lead to many other physical and mental health benefits as well.

We probably begin to learn to marginalize in childhood, and the marginalization continues unabated into our golden years. When the time for retirement arrives, many retirees are left with nothing to occupy their time. Recreation sounds good when you work every day, but once it becomes forced—once one is left with nothing else to do—it can become extremely stressful.

Children's lives are becoming increasingly marginalized as well. After school, many kids go to organized play or sports, arranged day care, or lessons of some sort, such as piano, gymnastics, and ballet. Little time is left for free play.

Entire households are falling prey to marginalized living. In over 65 percent of homes, both parents work. At the end of the day, these parents come home to another full-time job: making dinner, raising children, walking the dog, and so forth. In many marginalized homes, weeks go by without a single meal at which every family member is at the table eating and talking over the day's or week's events. Meals are often purchased from fast-food outlets and eaten on the run.

Problems with excess weight and obesity invariably accompany such fast-food diets because such foods are usually high in fat and dense in calories and come in larger-than-average portions. Add to that the lack of time in marginalized lives for exercise and active recreation, and you've got all the ingredients necessary for the health problems discussed in chapters 9 and 10, IBS among them.

THE NECESSITY OF DOWNTIME

Marginalization is not inherently bad; history has proven that some people seem to thrive on eighteen-hour workdays. Henry Kissinger, for example, flourished on four hours of sleep a day and could keep two shifts of assistants working. If you have IBS, however, such a lifestyle is not recommended.

People require downtime to relax and watch the grass grow or smell the roses. Downtime allows your subconscious mind to sift through things and reach conclusions. Experts call this process *mental digestion,* and most people require a good portion of it not only to find solutions to daily challenges but to maintain their grip on reality. Many individuals need to come home in the evening and simply relax, watch TV, read, pursue a hobby, or help kids with homework.

Assess the twenty-four hours you have in each day. Ask yourself what basic pleasures you really like and need. You might find that simply tending your garden is enough to restore your spirit, or you may prefer a nice hike, attending lectures on esoteric subjects, sketching or painting, or other easily pursued, pleasurable activities.

15

Reduce Stress with Herbs

A number of herbs have been touted as stress relievers. As we've learned, stress and IBS are closely linked, so stress-relieving herbs may indirectly help improve IBS as well. Medical research has shown that some herbs work very well and some don't work at all; the majority remain untested. If an herb is effective, it provides one or more physiologically active substances that relieve a symptom or cure an illness. These physiologically active substances probably have unwanted side effects just like modern drugs, many of which are derived from herbs. And as with drugs, a person can become dependent on an herb, experiencing withdrawal symptoms when the herb is no longer taken. So be sure to use caution when taking these or any other herbs. Be particularly careful and check with your doctor before taking herbs if you are using medication or are pregnant.

VALERIAN

Valerian root was probably the first human tranquilizer (after alcohol) and its original discovery is lost in the fog of prehistory. Valerian has been used for at least a thousand years to help people calm down and cope with what modern society calls stress. It was listed in the *United States Pharmacopoeia* from 1850 to 1940.

Valerian's active biochemicals attach themselves to the same sites in the brain that are affected by modern tranquilizers and mood elevators that are commonly prescribed for stress and anxiety. Animal and human research indicates that valerian helps people deal with stress and the anxiety that accompanies it.

Dosages of herbs can be problematic because herbs are not standardized as medications and vitamins are. Methods of preparation are also not standardized. So, even if the herb you're using has been tested and proven to be effective, the herb you purchase is probably not exactly the same as the one tested. Consequently, it might not deliver the expected effect. The efficacy of valerian varies with the method of preparation. Daily use should not exceed 15 grams of the plant material. That translates to:

- 15 to 20 drops of a 1:5 tincture in water two or three times daily;
- 1 teaspoon of root steeped 10 minutes in hot water, three times daily; or
- 1 tablespoon of valerian juice three times daily.

There are a few precautions:

- Pregnant women should not use valerian.
- Valerian may cause frequent urination.
- Use caution when operating machinery while taking valerian.
- Never use valerian when taking Ativan, Valium, or Xanax. Ask your pharmacist about possible interactions with other drugs.

KAVA

Kava is a muscle relaxant and antianxiety herb that has been clinically tested and proven effective. Kava has been used as a relaxant for hundreds, if not thousands, of years in Polynesia. Because there is no written record of the ancient history of this area, no one can say exactly when its use began. It is often called kava-kava, and the names are used interchangeably.

Clinical studies have actually tested kava against prescription antianxiety medications with reasonably comparable results. It's clearly an herb that works.

A daily dosage of about 200 milligrams of kava can be spread over three daily doses of about 65 milligrams each. The actual amount will vary according to the source, so take a 40- to 70-milligram dose three times daily and see if it helps you over a period of stress and anxiety. As with any substance used by a person with IBS, be sure to test the preparation with a food that you know does not cause you gastric trouble.

Kava, like most herbs, has not been tested for safety in either large quantities or normal use over long periods of time. It has never been tested in people with IBS. Its widespread use over hundreds of years, however, amounts to millions of man-years of use, with few reports of side effects. Of course, kava is a physiologically active relaxant, so be cautious when using it, as you would be with alcohol or any psychoactive medication.

Kava also comes with certain precautions:

- Kava should not be used by pregnant or nursing mothers.
- People with depression should avoid using kava.
- Don't use kava if driving or operating complex equipment.
- Don't mix kava with alcohol.
- Don't combine kava with drugs such as Ativan, Valium, or Xanax, or other sedative herbs, such as valerian.
- Kava should not be taken for a period of more than three months.

GINSENG

Ginseng has been employed as a tonic to counteract stress and improve health for over two thousand years. Since its use probably predates the first Asian medical writings, a safe bet would place ginseng as being actively used for over twenty-five hundred years. Although ginseng's exact mechanism remains elusive to modern medical science, its extensive use over two millenniums suggests it has some beneficial effects; otherwise, people would have simply stopped taking it.

Chinese medicine classifies ginseng as an *adaptogen*. This classification doesn't comply with any standard definition in Western medicine, so there is some understandable confusion about its effects. The Chinese herbalist-physician would say that ginseng works best when a person is stressed to his limits, by allowing him to better adapt to his environment. Based on that description, ginseng seems tailor-made for our complex, competitive, and stressful society.

This indication makes sense in view of some clinical studies of ginseng and its many components, which include a number of active compounds called *ginsenosides.* Either ginseng itself or specific ginsenosides have been shown to elicit the following physiological effects:

- Lowers blood pressure.
- Improves reaction to visual and auditory stimuli.
- Improves oxygen utilization during physical exercise.
- Reduces heart rate in physical exercise.
- Improves work output.
- Improves aerobic capacity.
- Improves mood and outlook.

The above list suggests that ginseng is a stimulant (improves alertness) under some conditions and a relaxant (lowers blood pressure) under other conditions; adaptogen seems an appropriate description, indeed.

In China, Korea, and Japan, ginseng is used in tea, as it is most effectively employed everywhere. In the United States, you can purchase ginseng pills, capsules, and even candies. There is absolutely no proof that these forms work, so experience must be your personal guide with these products. When using any herb that has a history as rich as ginseng's, however, it makes sense to follow traditional use and take it as a tea. Ginseng tea is quite pleasant and simply taking the time to drink it will have a calming effect. (Remember that with IBS you should approach any substance cautiously and test it to be sure that it does not cause a flare-up.) Take ½ teaspoon (1.75 grams) dried ginseng root in a cup of boiling water twice daily. Most experts recommend drinking ginseng tea for at least three weeks; others recommend drinking it for up to three months.

If taking ginseng in tablet, capsule, or powder form, it is important to follow the directions that come with these preparations. As with the tea, regular use of three weeks to three months is required for ginseng's effectiveness to fully emerge; take a smaller dose regularly rather than a large dose just once or twice.

Ginseng comes with the following precautions:

- Pregnant women, people with diabetes, or people on medication should consult their doctors before taking ginseng.
- People taking Coumadin or other anticoagulant medications should exercise caution or avoid taking ginseng.

16

Eat a Balanced Diet

A balanced diet is essential to good health. No matter what medication you're taking or what strategies you're employing to curb your IBS, you must eat a healthy diet. Eighty-five percent of all illnesses clear up with a good diet, exercise, rest, and stress reduction. Follow the proactive, protective eating plan presented in this chapter and you will feel better within a week. Your IBS symptoms may not completely disappear, but they'll most definitely improve. You'll sleep more soundly and get up with more bounce in the morning. If you're overweight, you'll lose weight. Within a month people will notice that you look better. As an added bonus, your risk of cancer and heart disease will diminish, and chances are good that you'll live longer.

THE BASIC DIET

Fruits and Vegetables

Get at least five servings of fruits and vegetables daily; nine servings are better.

One serving of fruit would be a medium apple, orange, pear, or similar fruit; three small plums or apricots; one-eighth of a large cantaloupe; half a small melon; or a 1-inch slice of watermelon.

A serving of vegetables is ½ cup if the vegetables are cooked, 1 cup if raw. For example, one serving would be a single, large stalk of broccoli, including the florets; six medium asparagus spears; two potatoes without skin or one baked potato with skin; or one medium-sized raw carrot.

Four rules apply when eating fruits and vegetables:

1. Eat one serving of deep green or dark red vegetables, such as spinach, broccoli, sweet red peppers, or carrots, daily.
2. Eat one serving of fruit raw, such as an orange, apple, or banana, daily.
3. Eat three servings of beans weekly, such as lima, red kidney, or lentils. Change varieties regularly.
4. Eat one serving of a mixed green salad with tomatoes and onions daily.

Grains and Cereals

Eat at least four servings of grains and cereals daily; six servings is ideal.

One cereal serving would be ⅓ cup of cold or cooked cereal; try to eat cereals that provide 4 or more grams of fiber per serving. For one serving of bread, eat one slice of whole-grain bread. One serving of pasta would be 1 cup if cooked, 2 ounces if dry. One serving of grains would be ½ cup of cooked grains such as rice or millet.

Eat one daily serving of high-fiber, natural cereal with low-fat or nonfat milk. Try to eat three varieties of high-fiber cereals weekly.

Natural Bulbs

Eat at least one serving of garlic, onions, leeks, shallots, or chives daily; more is better. Determining the serving size of natural bulbs is not as precise as for other vegetables, so simply try to work these bulbs into your diet as much as possible. For example, add one clove of garlic to flavor a salad, soup, meat, spaghetti sauce, and so on; add a quarter of an onion to your salad or vegetables; or mix ¼ cup chopped raw leeks into a dish. Flavor your foods with these bulbs regularly. You can't get too much.

Milk and Dairy Products

Eat three servings of low-fat dairy foods daily.

One cup of milk equals a serving. For yogurt, a serving is 6 ounces. For one serving of cheese, eat about 1½ ounces, or 40 grams.

Although ice cream is a dairy product, it requires 1 full pint to fulfill the nutritional requirements of one serving of dairy. Frozen yogurt is somewhat better because it contains fewer calories, but one serving still calls for 1 full pint. Newer low-fat ice creams are better yet, but be sure to read nutritional labels.

Protein-Rich Foods

Eat two servings of protein-rich foods daily.

For fish, poultry, and other meats, one serving equals 3½ ounces, about ¼ pound. (Don't eat processed meats, such as bologna or hot dogs.) Two medium eggs equal one serving. One serving of cheese is 1½ ounces. One serving of beans is 1 cup of cooked beans.

Every week, be sure to:

- Eat fish at least three times; two of those servings should be finfish.
- Eat one vegetarian meal; for example, eggs, beans, or pasta with cheese.
- Eat poultry as often as desired; just be sure to remove the skin after cooking.
- Eat red meat no more than once (see chapter 23 to learn about the difference between healthy and unhealthy oils).

Oils and Fats

For frying, use peanut oil, olive oil, or butter. Don't use safflower oil or other oil high in polyunsaturated fats. For baking, use canola oil or rapeseed oil. To dress salads, use cold-pressed olive oil, canola, walnut, avocado, or linseed oils.

Add 1 teaspoon of flaxseed oil daily to salad dressings or use in baking to increase your intake of the omega-3 oils. For some people, 1 to 3 tablespoons may be recommended. (See chapter 23 for more about the omega-3 oils.)

Water

Drink four 8-ounce glasses of water daily. Use purified water, mineral water, or distilled water. Seek out water that is free of nitrates, chlorides, and man-made chemicals, such as pesticides. Natural minerals, including calcium, magnesium, and so on, are a plus.

IMPROVING ON THE BASIC DIET

I encourage you to build on and improve this diet. If you become a fish-eating near-vegetarian, in contrast to the typical meat-eating American who eats 3 to 4.5 ounces of beef daily, you'll accelerate the benefits of the diet and will feel better sooner.

Think of your body as a castle and your diet as its foundation. Although scientists continue to argue over the merits of megadosing on vitamins and minerals, there's unanimous agreement that a few easy nutritional additions will pay huge health dividends. For example:

- Up to nine servings of fruits and vegetables daily are better than the basic five.

- Fish four or five times weekly is better than three; and no red meat is even better than some.
- Extra cruciferous vegetables and foods from the garlic family will add to the benefits of the diet.
- A high-fiber bran cereal is an excellent start for every day. Oat bran, wheat bran, rice bran, and corn bran are excellent for variety.
- An extra serving of beans prepared without fat will help reduce cholesterol and the risk of all the illnesses discussed in this book.
- Sensible supplementation will help.

Developing a few new habits can make the diet even more effective. You've probably heard these tips before, but they're worth repeating:

- Eat fruit for dessert; for example, a slice of melon, half a mango, or a slice of watermelon.
- Snack on vegetables, fruit, and nuts.
- Always use whole-grain breads or rolls.
- Drink an 8-ounce glass of water first thing in the morning, thirty minutes before each meal, and once before bedtime.

MENUS

Following are seven daily food plans I have developed to illustrate the diet's versatility. In a number of instances, I have included a calorie breakdown to give you a feeling for caloric quantities. Make a game out of designing imaginative and varied menus of your own. (For a good guide to alternatives to various foods, I recommend *Bowes & Church's Food Values of Portions Commonly Used*, 15th ed., by Jean A. T. Pennington, Ph.D., R.D.)

Day 1	

Meal	Calories
Breakfast	
Glass of water	
½ grapefruit	39
All-Bran cereal	70
with low-fat milk (104 calories), ½ sliced banana (52 calories)	156
1 slice whole-grain bread, toasted (61 calories) and buttered (36 calories)	97
Tea or coffee (optional)	
Midmorning Snack	
Glass of water	
Peach yogurt	260
Lunch	
Glass of water	
Bean soup	157
1 whole-wheat roll (72 calories) with butter (36 calories)	108
Lettuce salad (4 calories) with tomatoes (12 calories),	
cucumber (4 calories), green pepper (5 calories), and onions (4 calories),	
Italian dressing (14 calories)	43
Lime sherbet	135
Tea or coffee (optional)	
Afternoon Snack	
Glass of water	
Apple (81 calories) with cheddar cheese (114 calories)	195
Dinner	
Glass of water	
Broiled salmon with herbs	100
Baked potato (88 calories) with sour cream and chives (26 calories)	114
Steamed broccoli	12
Low-fat ice cream (140 calories) with sliced strawberries (22 calories)	162
Tea or coffee (optional)	
Evening Snack	
Pear	98
Day 1 Total	**1746**

Day 2

Meal	Calories
Breakfast	
Glass of water	
Slice of cantaloupe	57
Oatmeal (109 calories) with raisins (56 calories),	
low-fat milk (104 calories)	269
Whole-wheat English muffin (170 calories) with butter (36 calories)	206
Tea or coffee (optional)	
Midmorning Snack	
Glass of water	
Bran muffin	112
Lunch	
Glass of water	
Tuna fish salad (172 calories) sandwich on	
whole-wheat bread (122 calories)	294
Carrot sticks	31
Coleslaw	42
Tea or coffee (optional)	
Afternoon Snack	
Glass of water	
Pear (98 calories) with feta cheese (75 calories)	173
Dinner	
Glass of water	
Cheese ravioli with tomato sauce with onions, garlic, spices	284
Mixed salad greens (5 calories), with tomatoes (12 calories),	
green pepper (5 calories), garbanzo beans (32 calories),	
Italian dressing (14 calories)	68
Cannoli	171
Tea or coffee (optional)	
Evening Snack	
Apple	81
Day 2 Total	**1788**

Day 3

Meal	Calories
Breakfast	
Glass of water	
Orange-grapefruit juice	80
Sliced oranges and strawberries	55
Whole-wheat waffles (206 calories) with maple syrup (50 calories)	256
Tea or coffee (optional)	
Midmorning Snack	
Glass of water	
Cheddar cheese (114 calories) and grapes (75 calories)	189
Lunch	
Glass of water	
Salmon quiche	215
Triple-bean salad	90
Pear	98
Tea or coffee (optional)	
Afternoon Snack	
Glass of water	
Carrot and celery sticks	35
Dinner	
Glass of water	
Wok chicken (202 calories) with broccoli (12 calories), red peppers (12 calories), onion (6 calories), garlic, ginger, and mushrooms (20 calories)	252
Rice	112
Mixed green salad (5 calories) with water chestnuts (15 calories), green onions (7 calories), and mandarin oranges (23 calories), Thousand Island dressing (24 calories)	74
Apple-tapioca pudding	101
Tea or coffee (optional)	
Evening Snack	
Banana	105
Day 3 Total	**1662**

Day 4

Meal	Calories
Breakfast	
Glass of water	
Slice of melon (57 calories) with blueberries (41 calories)	98
2 poached eggs (158 calories) on whole-wheat toast (63 calories)	221
1 slice lean ham	50
Tea or coffee (optional)	
Midmorning Snack	
Glass of water	
Blueberry muffin	176
Lunch	
Glass of water	
Curried chicken salad on lettuce	136
Banana bread	85
Frozen banana yogurt	143
Tea or coffee (optional)	
Afternoon Snack	
Glass of water	
Grapes	58
Dinner	
Glass of water	
Halibut steak, broiled	119
Mixed green salad (5 calories) with tomatoes (12 calories), onions (7 calories), red pepper (6 calories), zesty tomato dressing (11 calories)	41
Carrots	31
Asparagus	12
Rice	112
Apple strudel	96
Tea or coffee (optional)	
Evening Snack	
Brick cheese (105 calories) and whole-wheat crackers (70 calories)	175
Pear	98
Day 4 Total	**1651**

Day 5

Meal	Calories
Breakfast	
Glass of water	
Sliced oranges, bananas, and kiwi fruit	72
Fiber One cereal (60 calories) with low-fat milk (104 calories)	164
Bran muffin (112 calories), with butter (36 calories)	148
Tea or coffee (optional)	
Midmorning Snack	
Glass of water	
Fruit yogurt	260
Lunch	
Glass of water	
Lentil soup	69
Melted cheese (96 calories) and crab (74 calories) on	
English muffin (68 calories)	238
Mixed salad greens (5 calories) with tomatoes (12 calories),	
cucumbers (4 calories), zesty tomato dressing (11 calories)	32
Pear	98
Tea or coffee (optional)	
Afternoon Snack	
Glass of water	
Celery sticks (12 calories) with peanut butter (47 calories)	59
Carrot sticks	31
Dinner	
Glass of water	
Zucchini lasagna with tomato sauce with onions, garlic, and herbs	189
Corn	89
Lemon, cabbage, carrot mold with lettuce	57
Crusty French bread, butter	81
Cheesecake	150
Tea or coffee (optional)	
Evening Snack	
Plum	36
Day 5 Total	**1773**

Day 6

Meal	Calories
Breakfast	
Glass of water	
½ papaya	59
Fiber One cereal (60 calories) with low-fat milk (104 calories) and blueberries (41 calories)	205
Tea or coffee (optional)	
Midmorning Snack	
Glass of water	
Fruit yogurt	260
Lunch	
Glass of water	
Spinach salad (56 calories) with mushrooms (40 calories), chopped egg (40 calories), onion (27 calories), bacon bits (21 calories), oil, vinegar, and mustard dressing (34 calories)	218
Popover	90
Sliced peaches	66
Tea or coffee (optional)	
Afternoon Snack	
Glass of water	
Rice cakes (35 calories) with cream cheese (98 calories)	133
Dinner	
Glass of water	
Filet of sole	80
Basil bean salad with onions, garlic	90
Rice pilaf	121
Spinach	6
Pumpkin pie	212
Tea or coffee (optional)	
Evening Snack	
Pear	98
Day 6 Total	**1638**

Day 7

Meal	Calories
Breakfast	
Glass of water	
Sliced peaches (37 calories) with low-fat cottage cheese (41 calories)	78
Whole-wheat pancakes (142 calories) with blueberries (41 calories)	
and maple syrup (50 calories)	233
Tea or coffee (optional)	
Midmorning Snack	
Glass of water	
Fruit yogurt	260
Lunch	
Glass of water	
Creamy carrot soup	149
Salmon salad with lettuce and tomato (110 calories) in	
half pita bread (53 calories)	163
Raspberries	61
Tea or coffee (optional)	
Afternoon Snack	
Glass of water	
Applesauce wheat bar	134
Dinner	
Glass of water	
Marinated lamb roast with garlic	180
Tossed greens (5 calories) with sliced canned pears (50 calories)	55
Small roasted potatoes	65
Green beans	22
Whole-wheat roll (72 calories) with butter (36 calories)	108
Lemon dream parfaits	176
Tea or coffee (optional)	
Evening Snack	
Orange	65
Day 7 Total	**1749**

Once, after I'd finished a lecture on dieting, a woman who'd been in the audience approached me and asked, "When do I start?" "Immediately," I answered. This, the first instant of the rest of your life, is the best time to begin developing eating habits that will help you live longer and help you live better.

17

Eat More Dietary Fiber

Health scientists have usually looked at IBS from several vantage points: as a dietary fiber problem, as a food sensitivity, as a psychologically related condition, or as some combination of all three. Each approach has had positive results, so be a pragmatist and make use of each. We've already discussed the roles of food sensitivity and psychology in IBS in previous chapters; in this chapter we'll examine the part fiber plays in controlling IBS.

Many modern health problems in addition to IBS are in part due to the decline in the amount and type of dietary fiber we get from our food. This decline parallels the increase in industrialization and has accelerated in recent decades with the proliferation of processed foods and convenience eating. Because we live longer now, the cumulative effects of fiber deficiency have more time to develop, and they tend to show up as we get older. This makes fiber deficiency particularly insidious because its results don't emerge until it's too late to apply correct dietary measures. Prevention is indeed the best medicine for fiber deficiency.

Answer the following questions:

- Are your bowel movements irregular (for example, you don't have a bowel movement with firm, light brown stools once every twenty-four to thirty-six hours)?

- Have you or a blood relative ever had gallstones or gallbladder disease?
- Have you or a blood relative ever had diverticulosis, hemorrhoids, appendicitis, or varicose veins in the thighs?
- If you're over the age of thirty-five, is your total cholesterol less than 200 milligrams per deciliter of blood? Is your HDL cholesterol over 50 milligrams per deciliter?
- Have you or any blood relative ever had cancer of the colon or rectum, or polyps?

If you answered yes to any of these questions, increasing your dietary fiber could have a profound effect on your health.

WHAT IS DIETARY FIBER?

Dietary fiber is the indigestible part of plant-based foods; it passes through the stomach and small intestine without being digested. Plant-based foods come in an incredible variety of fruits, vegetables, and edible flowers, from spinach, to red and bulgur wheat, to Delicious and Macintosh apples, to kidney and pinto beans. Each variety provides its own unique dietary fiber.

There are six general types of dietary fiber, with hard, insoluble bran at one extreme and gums at the other (see Table 17.1). Plant cell walls are a matrix of these six types of fiber; the specific makeup varies from plant to plant. Most plants contain some or all of them, even though one type of fiber might dominate. For example, wheat grain has an outer coat of bran, or hard fiber, to withstand the elements and keep the content of the grain intact.

Our bodies have adapted to the availability and functions of each type of fiber. We depend on fiber just as we rely on vitamins. The body functions that call for fiber, however, are far more subtle than those that require vitamins, so our dependence on fiber isn't as obvious. A vitamin deficiency produces a well-defined set of symptoms

Table 17.1

The Six Types of Fiber

Fiber Type	Water-Soluble?	Function in Plant	Food Sources
Cellulose	No	Forms structure of cell walls with lignins	Wheat bran, fruit peels, seed coats
Lignin	No	Forms structure of cell walls with cellulose	Cereal grains, potato skins
Hemicellulose	Partly	Holds cells together with cellulose	Wheat bran, grains
Pectin	Yes	Binds cells together and holds water in fruit	Fruits
Gum	Yes	Binds stems, seeds, and vegetables	Oatmeal, legumes, vegetables
Mucilages	Yes	Binds seeds; binds stems in aquatic plants	Seaweed, seeds

in a month or so. Restore the vitamin and the symptoms start to disappear in hours, if not a few days. In contrast, a fiber deficiency may start in childhood, and show up as diverticulosis or hemorrhoids at age forty or fifty. By then, it's too late to address the cause of the illness. Taking fiber when you have diverticulosis can relieve the symptoms but can't reverse the damage that has been done.

During the 1960s, Dr. Hugh Trowell and Dr. Dennis Burkitt, medical missionaries to South Africa, noticed that there were startling health differences in the incidence of intestinal diseases between urban city dwellers and rural people. They also observed differences between black and white populations. These differences, correlated with the amount of fiber in each group's diet, are listed in Table 17.2.

There's no longer any doubt among scientists that fiber is the most important nutrient in regard to bowel-related diseases. It plays an important part in many other modern illnesses as well:

- Cancer. Fiber detoxifies dietary and metabolic factors, helping prevent colorectal and stomach cancer, as well as cancers in which bowel regularity is important, such as stomach, pancreatic, breast, and prostate cancer.

Table 17.2

Noninfective Bowel Diseases in South African Populations

	Rural Blacks (never lived in urban areas)	Urban Blacks (raised in rural areas)	Urban Whites (never lived in rural areas)
Dietary fiber, grams consumed per day	40 or more	25 or more	17 or less
Fiber-Related Illnesses			
Hemorrhoids	rare	++	+++
Appendicitis	+	++	+++++
Ulcerative colitis	rare	+	+++++
IBS	+	++	++++
Diverticular disease	rare	+	+++++
Colon cancer	rare	+	+++++

Note: The rate at which an illness appears is indicated by the symbol +, with one + indicating that the illness was seen occasionally, and +++++ indicating that the illness was a serious cause of death or debilitation.

Source: These data are taken from many research papers. For a review, see A. R. P. Walker and I. Segal, "Epidemiology of Noninfective Bowel Diseases in South African Populations," *Tropical Gastroenterology* 4, no. 155 (1983).

- Heart disease. A high-fiber diet is a low-fat diet, which helps prevent elevated blood fats such as cholesterol and triglycerides, as well as high blood pressure.
- Intestinal disorders. Fiber helps to tone the intestine, combating gallbladder disease, ileitis, colitis and ulcerative colitis, appendicitis, inflammatory bowel diseases, diverticulosis, varicose veins, and hemorrhoids.
- Diabetes. A high-fiber diet is a low-sugar diet, which helps with the reduction and stabilization of blood sugar.

HOW FIBER WORKS

Fiber is like a brush with selective bristles that, in addition to moving things along, can selectively bind unwanted materials and remove them from the system. Each of the six types of fiber has specific properties we require. Of course, selective supplementation helps (see chapter 18).

Hard fiber, the type found in wheat bran, is the water carrier that helps to produce regularity. It gives stools consistency. This fiber is found in all plant food but mostly in the high-fiber cereals, grains, most vegetables, beans, and tubers such as potatoes. You can't eat too much of these foods, and the results will be obvious as you increase them in your diet.

In contrast to the hard fiber, the soluble forms of fiber, such as pectin, gums, saponins, and others, are the best at selective absorption. For example, pectin helps to reduce cholesterol by binding the bile acids produced by our livers from cholesterol and removing them in our stools. Oat bran does it even better, and guar gum better yet. Soluble fiber also binds the cholesterol and fat that we get in our diet and helps to carry them through the system.

The two most important functions of dietary fiber are to bulk the stools, making them firm and easy to move, and preventing them from being watery; and to bind unwanted materials. Fiber's ability to bind water makes it a key element in preventing diarrhea, and its ability to bind bile acid helps prevent pain and irritation in the lower colon and around the anus—good news for IBS sufferers!

GETTING THE FIBER YOU NEED FROM FOOD

How much fiber is enough? Extensive research has proven that, for optimal bowel function, the body needs about 25 to 40 grams of fiber daily. I recommend that people aim for 35 grams. About two-thirds of that amount should be hard or insoluble fiber and the remaining third should be soft or soluble fiber. Getting enough correctly balanced fiber prevents watery or hard stools and produces firm but soft, easily moved stools. When you're getting the right amount and right mix of fiber, you'll move light brown stools once every twenty-four to thirty-six hours, and more likely every twenty-four hours or less.

An easy way to get a good start on the fiber you need is to begin each day with high-fiber cereal. Many excellent cereals are available: Fiber One, All-Bran, Bran Buds, bran flakes, corn bran, oat bran, oatmeal, and barley, to name a few. Add unprocessed bran to pancakes or waffles. Eat fruit on cereal, in pancakes, or alone; eat fruit and more fruit along with vegetables, grains, and tubers at each meal. As your fiber intake improves, you'll become more regular. Table 17.3 contains some readily available cereals that provide sufficient dietary fiber.

Fiber and Water

Water is essential to fiber's effectiveness. Since fiber is the plant material that binds water, it can bind *you* up if you don't get enough water. In the presence of water, fiber makes your stools soft and consistent; in the absence of water, it can make them dry and hard.

Table 17.3

Fiber from Cereals

Fiber per Serving	Cereals	
(g)	**Cold**	**Hot**
3–5	Quaker Corn Bran	Quaker Oats
	Ralston Bran Chex	Malt-O-Meal
		Hot Wheat Cereal
	Kellogg's Raisin Bran	Ralston Cream of Wheat
	Generic/store brand	Wheatena
	raisin bran	
	Kellogg's Cracklin' Oat Bran	Unprocessed bran
	Kellogg's Bran Flakes	Miller unprocessed bran
	General Mills Raisin	Quaker unprocessed bran
	Nut Bran	
	Post Fruit 'N Fiber	
	Post Bran Flakes	
	Post Natural Raisin Bran	
9	Kellogg's All-Bran	
	Nabisco 100% Bran	
Over 12	Kellogg's All-Bran	
	Extra Fiber	
	General Mills Fiber One	

Our requirement for water extends far beyond its relationship to fiber, of course. Indeed, next to air itself, it is the most important of all nutrients. In IBS it is especially important for the elimination of waste materials that, in the opinion of some experts, can cause flare-ups.

Strive to consume eight glasses of water daily, preferably as pure water rather than in the form of other beverages.

Table 17.4

A Day with 35 Grams of Fiber

Food Item	Soluble	Insoluble	Total	Calories
Breakfast				
Bran flakes	1.0	4.0	5.0	121
(with ½ cup skim milk)				93
½ grapefruit	0.6	1.1	1.7	39
Snack				
Banana	0.6	1.4	2.0	105
Lunch				
2 slices wheat bread	0.6	2.2	2.8	122
Corn (½ cup)	1.7	2.2	3.9	89
Broccoli	1.6	2.3	3.9	23
Peach (dessert)	0.6	1.0	1.6	37
Snack				
Apple	0.8	2.0	2.8	81
Dinner				
Brussels sprouts	1.6	2.3	3.9	30
Small salad	1.6	2.2	3.8	50
Potato	0.7	1.0	1.7	200
Melon (dessert)	0.4	0.6	1.0	130
Snack				
Pear (crispy)	0.5	2.0	2.5	98
Total	**12.3**	**24.3**	**36.6**	**1218**

Other foods eaten during the day	Calories
Yogurt, low-fat	228
Fish	150
Turkey slices	100
Spreads and condiments	100
Total calories	**578**
Total daily calories	**1796**

Note: This day is designed to provide enough fiber with flexibility. There's room to have other desserts or accompaniments, such as wine, up to 1,800 calories for women and 2,200 calories for men.

A DAY WITH 35 GRAMS OF FIBER

Some people have difficulty understanding how taking in 25 to 35 grams of fiber daily is accomplished, so I've prepared Table 17.4. This "Day of Fiber" exceeds what most people require; for example, a 125-pound woman may do fine on 25 to 30 grams daily, while a 200-pound man may need 35 grams.

These guidelines allow for many substitutions. For instance, beans and rice would be an excellent protein entrée that also provides fiber. That combination could easily substitute for a luncheon sandwich.

You cannot get too much dietary fiber. In the past thirty years, I've never observed a study in which people have gotten too much dietary fiber, and that includes those in which the volunteers took 90 grams daily.

18

Can't Eat Cereal?
Try Fiber Supplements

You may find that eating cereal in the morning causes your IBS to flare up. You should still consume 25 to 35 grams of dietary fiber daily, as recommended in chapter 17; you will simply have to use a fiber supplement to do so. Fiber is too essential to good health—particularly GI health—to go without.

Even if cereal isn't a problem for you, you may want to consider taking a daily fiber supplement. Many studies on modern diets confirm that most people do not get the recommended 25 to 35 grams of dietary fiber daily. In fact, the average person's diet falls below 13 grams daily. That means most people are eating a diet that provides less than 50 percent of their daily fiber needs. For some, achieving the daily fiber requirement, with or without a high-fiber cereal, may be nearly impossible without the use of a fiber supplement.

Metamucil sets the standard for fiber supplements and has several advantages for IBS patients: it is highly refined, so the rough edges of the psyllium husks used in most fiber supplements are unlikely to cause discomfort; in addition, because Metamucil is highly purified, it is less likely to ferment in the lower GI tract, resulting in less gas production and flatulence.

Most drugstore chains sell their own private-label fiber supplements. These store and other brands are usually sold as "natural fiber laxatives," "natural fiber supplements," or simply "psyllium." Because they are often less expensive than Metamucil, you may want to try them—carefully, of course, as you would with any food.

Fiber supplements work best when taken with meals. After all, fiber is normally part of food, so it belongs with food. It can be taken anywhere from thirty minutes before to thirty minutes after a meal. A good approach is to take a tablespoon of fiber supplement in water with each meal, and one more either in between meals or after dinner. Always take fiber at least thirty minutes before going to bed.

TREATING IBS SYMPTOMS WITH FIBER SUPPLEMENTS

Extensive clinical studies of fiber used as a supplement prove that it stops diarrhea and also stops constipation. When you have diarrhea, a simple approach is to take a rounded tablespoon of fiber dissolved in water after each movement. It will take some time for the fiber to work, but eventually it will stop the diarrhea as well as eliminate the irritation that often accompanies it.

If you take either prescription or nonprescription medication for diarrhea, you can still take your fiber supplement. Not only will it produce regularity, but it will generally make the medication more effective; you'll probably be able to get along with less.

ADDED BENEFITS
Weight Loss

A simple trick used by dieters is to take a fiber supplement about twenty to thirty minutes before mealtime. This will make you feel full, or satiated, and you will eat less. Fiber supplements used in this manner will make just about any weight-loss diet work more effectively.

Reducing Cholesterol

As we discussed in chapter 17, fiber binds bile acids. Binding bile acids indirectly lowers cholesterol. Fiber supplements taken four times daily will generally lower blood cholesterol by about 10 percent, a very significant amount and a clear improvement in health.

19

Take a Basic Multiple Vitamin and Mineral Supplement Daily

To function normally, your body—including your GI tract—requires nineteen vitamins and minerals daily in addition to protein, fat, carbohydrates, and fiber. These requirements are expressed as a recommended daily intake (RDI). Vitamins and most minerals are required in very small (trace) quantities. For example, every day you need just 400 micrograms (400 millionths of a gram) of the B vitamin folic acid. In contrast, calcium is required in comparatively large amounts, ranging from 1,000 milligrams (1 gram) for most women up to about age fifty to 1,200 milligrams for those over fifty. The requirement for magnesium is somewhat midway; you need 200 to 400 milligrams (⅖ of a gram) daily. With the exception of calcium and magnesium (which are discussed in detail in chapter 20), all your vitamin and mineral needs can be packed into a single tablet. I don't believe in leaving anything to chance, so I recommend that you supplement your diet to avoid any possible marginal deficiencies.

Use a supplement that provides the vitamins and minerals in the amounts listed in Table 19.1. Most supplements will contain within 10 to 20 percent of the values listed here. It is important that your supplement contains all these vitamins and minerals and that you take it daily.

Few products satisfy these criteria completely. Usually the product you select will have less calcium and magnesium. If this is true, do not worry, because you should take extra calcium anyway. Your diet already contains excess phosphorus and about 20 percent of the magnesium you need. If the supplement you choose comes within 20 percent of the calcium, magnesium, and phosphorus listed in Table 19.1, it is fine. Don't select a supplement that varies in these three areas by more than that amount.

IS MORE BETTER?

Most vitamins are safe at ten or more times the RDI, so if you choose to take a multivitamin that provides some extra, you don't have to worry; you're not harming yourself. Recent studies of elderly people indicate that as we get older our needs increase, so taking more than the RDI is undoubtedly a good idea if you're over the age of fifty.

COMMON QUESTIONS ABOUT SUPPLEMENT USE

Question: Aren't excess vitamins and minerals just excreted, making expensive urine?
Answer: Even if you're starving, your body will lose some vitamins and minerals daily through excretion. Under those conditions, your urine is truly "expensive." If your blood levels of nutrients are high, your urine levels will also be higher; that is normal human physiology.

Table 19.1

Basic Supplements

Nutrient Vitamin	Amount per Tablet*	Percent U.S. RDI
Vitamin A (as beta carotene)	2,500 I.U.** (500 mcg RE***)	50
Vitamin D	200 I.U. (5 mcg)	50
Vitamin E	15 I.U. (5 mg alpha-tocopherol equivalents)	50
Vitamin C	30 mg	50
Folic acid	0.2 mg	50
Thiamin (B_1)	0.75 mg	50
Riboflavin (B_2)	0.86 mg	50
Niacin	10 mg	50
Vitamin B_6	1 mg	50
Vitamin B_{12}	3 mcg	50
Biotin	0.15 mg (150 mcg)	50
Pantothenic acid	5 mg	50

Nutrient Mineral

Calcium	125 mg	25
Phosphorus	180 mg	40
Iodine	75 mcg	50
Iron	9 mg	50
Magnesium	50 mg	12.5
Copper	1 mg	50
Zinc	1 mg	50
Selenium	50 mcg	****
Manganese	0.5 mg	****
Chromium	50 mcg	****
Molybdenum	30 mcg	****

* Two tablets provide 100 percent U.S. RDI for all nutrients except calcium, phosphorus, and magnesium.
** International Units.
*** Microgram retinol equivalents.
**** U.S. RDI not established.

Question: Isn't it expensive to take vitamins and minerals?

Answer: Our society spends about $1.00 per capita daily on soft drinks. Is that wasteful? The average adult woman spends about $1.00 daily on her hair. Expensive is meaningful only by comparison. A multiple vitamin and mineral supplement costs less than 25 cents daily. Is your health worth 25 cents a day?

Question: A salesperson I know sells a brand of vitamins not available in stores. He says they're better and are all natural, but they're quite expensive. Should I use them?

Answer: Just about all basic vitamins sold as supplements are made by five companies worldwide. Every atom in each vitamin is as natural as the atom in any other vitamin, so there is no point in purchasing a product that purports to be all natural. My advice is to go with a good brand name, usually a major pharmaceutical firm, because these companies have the most to lose if something goes wrong. Besides, the quality control methods used by these manufacturers have been developed for the very quantitative pharmaceutical industry, so they are likely to be exact.

Question: I notice some companies have products that are targeted by age group. I understand supplements specifically designed for children, but what about those aimed at seniors?

Answer: If the product supplies at least what is called for in Table 19.1, it is fine. A little more won't hurt.

20

Get Enough Calcium and Magnesium

Obtaining sufficient calcium and magnesium from foods alone is difficult for people with no intestinal disorders and is a special nutritional challenge for people with IBS. People with IBS and other intestinal disorders are often lactose intolerant, so they can't digest milk sugar and often get diarrhea from dairy products. Hence, people with IBS learn to avoid dairy products.

Without dairy products, obtaining the recommended 1,000 to 1,500 milligrams of calcium daily solely from food is a major challenge for a dietician or nutritionist, let alone an average person with IBS. Even though calcium-fortified foods, such as orange juice, are available, a person should "take out insurance" by using calcium supplements.

Recent government nutrition and food analyses indicate that calcium is generally short in most young adults' and adults' diets. In fact, many experts both use and recommend calcium supplements. In addition to the difficulty IBS sufferers in particular face in obtaining adequate dietary calcium through calcium-rich foods, many lifestyle habits, such as caffeine, excess sodium, and lack of exercise, cause calcium loss. Therefore, common sense dictates that beginning at about age thirteen to fifteen, people should take 400 to 600 milligrams of calcium daily.

Unlike many nutrients, calcium shortfalls are additive. That means that if you fall short for a year or two, say, when you're a teenager, and then you do it again during your childbearing years as a mature adult, you will have less dense bones than if you hadn't fallen short at all. Below-normal bone density is a disease called *osteoporosis,* which causes much suffering and even death after age sixty-five.

Adult women require 1,000 milligrams of calcium each day up to about age fifty, and most health experts and nutritionists believe that their calcium intake should then be elevated to 1,200 or 1,500 milligrams. Milk, yogurt, and cheese are the most common sources of calcium; in contrast, a 1-cup serving of broccoli or spinach provides $\frac{1}{10}$ the calcium of a glass of milk. A cup of milk provides about 300 milligrams of calcium, as does a 6-ounce serving of yogurt and about 2 to 5 ounces of cheese. To get sufficient calcium from diet alone, you'd need about three glasses of milk daily, as well as four to five servings of deep green vegetables—not an easy proposition for the food sensitive.

Much emphasis is placed on women's calcium needs, but men could do well by following the same advice as that given to women. Because men don't have to bear children and have different hormones, they need about 60 to 80 percent of the calcium required by women. Past about age twenty-one, however, men tend to fall short in their calcium intake. Then, as they get older (say, at about age fifty), they need almost as much as women.

Bone calcium loss is accelerated by caffeine (coffee, tea, soft drinks), excess meat and salt, and inadequate exercise. Clinical research in many countries, however, has proven that bone density can be restored by using calcium supplements. If you drink more than two cups of coffee a day or its equivalent as tea or soft drinks, take an extra 200 milligrams daily.

MAGNESIUM: A PARTNER WITH CALCIUM

Most dietary analyses indicate that we usually do not get enough of the mineral magnesium as well as calcium. Since 200 to 400 milligrams of magnesium are required daily, it, like calcium, doesn't fit into a single tablet. A good policy is to take a calcium supplement that also contains some magnesium.

Some self-proclaimed experts advise a specific calcium/magnesium ratio for good health. A brilliant scientist, Dr. Mildred Seelig, conducted a careful study of adult needs for calcium and magnesium, however, and proved that once you achieve about 400 milligrams of magnesium daily, the body can use calcium very effectively and there is no need to ingest additional magnesium.

COMMON QUESTIONS ABOUT CALCIUM

Question: Will calcium cause kidney stones?

Answer: No! Extensive research in both men and women has proven that calcium actually reduces the risk of kidney stone formation. It is also essential to note that the same research indicated that a person who has a tendency toward stone formation should drink generous amounts of fluids.

Question: Should I take 1,000 to 1,500 milligrams of calcium at one time?

Answer: No, calcium will be absorbed more efficiently if you spread it over two or three doses daily. For example, if you take 1,200 milligrams daily, take 600 milligrams in the morning and 600 milligrams in the evening, or take 400 milligrams three times a day.

Question: When should I take calcium?

Answer: Calcium is absorbed best when it is taken with food. The carbohydrates in food seem to facilitate calcium absorption. So, take calcium supplements at mealtimes.

21

Increase Your Vitamin Intake: B Complex, C, and E

Basal metabolism (see chapter 9) accounts for most of the energy we use daily. In addition, people with IBS are often stressed by the condition, elevating their metabolism as part of their body's normal defense mechanism. Flare-ups produce yet more stress.

For metabolism to function smoothly, the body requires an adequate supply of the B vitamins, called *B complex*. These vitamins are often called "the stress vitamins" because people who are under stress seem to function better when they take these vitamins as supplements. (Some people with mild depression don't feel depressed when taking extra B-complex vitamins as well.) For these reasons, people with IBS should consider taking a balanced daily B-complex supplement and supplementing with vitamins C and E as well.

Taking a multiple vitamin and mineral supplement, as advised in chapter 19, should provide an adequate amount of all the necessary vitamins and minerals if you eat a fairly good diet. If you live or work in a stressful environment, however, or if you engage in active, aggressive, physical activity, more of the B-complex vitamins, as well as vitamins C and E, is required. Review your environment and decide for yourself:

- Do you live under stressful conditions?
- Do you work in a stressful environment?
- Do you commute over thirty minutes a day in heavy traffic?
- Are you exposed to a smoky or air-polluted environment?
- Are you exposed to solvent fumes?
- Do you take patented or prescription medication regularly?
- Do you engage in intense physical activity for over thirty minutes daily?

Answering yes to any of these questions could mean you need more of these nutrients, so read on.

B-COMPLEX VITAMINS

All metabolism requires the seven B vitamins, shown in Table 21.1.

Research has proven that when under physical stress and especially physical injury, the body needs more of these nutrients. When

Table 21.1

The B-Complex Vitamins

Vitamin	RDI
Thiamin (B_1)	1.5 mg
Riboflavin (B_2)	1.7 mg
Niacin	19 mg
Pyridoxal phosphate (B_6)	2.0 mg
B_{12}	2.0 mcg
Biotin	60 mcg
Folic acid	200 mcg

people are under emotional stress, they often feel more relaxed when they take extra B-complex vitamins.

Some experts call the B-complex vitamins *stress relievers,* and a number of physicians prescribe them to people who are under stress or feeling depressed. The simplest way to rule out B-complex deficiency as a factor in stress—and therefore in IBS—is to simply take an extra amount as a daily supplement.

If you take a B-complex supplement, make sure your supplement is balanced with the RDI given in Table 21.1.

VITAMIN C

Research suggests that the RDI of vitamin C should be about 100 to 150 milligrams under most conditions. If you live or work in a smoky environment or must commute long hours by car in heavy traffic, you need more vitamin C than indicated by the RDI. Both smoke and air pollution rob the body of vitamin C.

When your body is placed under stress, it uses more vitamin C to counter the attack and its vitamin C–level drops. The vitamin C–level in leukocytes, the white blood cells that are your body's first line of defense against infection, also drops, weakening the cells and allowing viruses to multiply. Vitamin C speeds the production of immune materials, which is why taking vitamin C makes a cold less severe.

You can get 100 to 500 milligrams of vitamin C daily by starting your morning with orange juice and then making sure you get at least four or more servings of fruits and vegetables.

People who regularly use aspirin or other nonsteroidal anti-inflammatory drugs (NSAIDs) or steroids require more vitamin C, an extra 500 milligrams daily. Even for people who don't meet these conditions, taking up to 1,000 milligrams of vitamin C daily will have some benefits and no negative side effects. If you decide to take a vitamin C supplement, select one that provides 500 milligrams per tablet. Should you decide you need 1,000 milligrams daily, take one 500-milligram tablet twice daily, in the morning and evening.

VITAMIN E

Age spots *(fleurs de cimitiere* in French) appear on the backs of our hands, on our faces, and on other parts of the body as we age. Although you can't see them, they also appear on the internal organs.

These spots are locations where pigments involving rancid oils, called lipofuscin, have accumulated. French folk wisdom holds that wheat germ or wheat germ oil prevents age spots. The only nutritional way to prevent the onset of age spots is with vitamin E, and wheat germ oil happens to be the best natural source of vitamin E. This folk wisdom goes right to the heart of vitamins E's function: preventing the oxidation of essential oils in the body. In this way, vitamin E actually slows the aging process.

If you want to get 50 milligrams of vitamin E daily, you will need to take a supplement that contains at least 30 milligrams, and you'd be better off taking one that provides 40 milligrams. One advantage of taking extra vitamin E is that it is retained by your body. Therefore, if you took a 400 IU supplement or 240 milligrams once weekly, that would maintain a running average of about 50 milligrams daily if you eat a good diet. Since almost all the most concentrated sources of vitamin E are very high in calories, a vitamin E supplement will more easily fit into a diet with healthy calorie limits than trying to obtain this much from food sources.

22

Maintain Healthy Potassium Levels

Diarrhea has one clear, undisputed side effect that people suffering from it are seldom told about: it causes the body to lose potassium. Potassium loss has many effects, from simple fatigue to serious heart problems in extreme cases. Potassium loss also upsets the body's K-factor (K-factor simply stands for the ratio of potassium to sodium). If prolonged over ten or more years, this imbalance is almost certain to cause high blood pressure. Anyone with IBS should get enough potassium and monitor dietary K-factor ratios.

In a natural diet, sodium and chloride, the components of common salt, are very scarce, and potassium is abundant. In fact, our kidneys conserve sodium and release potassium because of this. Salt is so abundant in affluent societies, however, that people sprinkle it on icy sidewalks and use it abundantly in most processed foods. This naturally leads to a lower potassium-to-sodium ratio, or K-factor, than that for which our bodies are designed. A correct K-factor cannot be restored by simply taking a potassium supplement because physiological problems in the GI tract are involved and the daily potassium requirement is quite high. Therefore, a commitment to an appropriate K-factor through diet is absolutely essential.

Table 22.1			
The K-Factor in Common Foods			
Food	**Sodium** **(mg per serving)**	**Potassium** **(mg per serving)**	**K-Factor**
Beef	44	311	7.00
Hot dog (all beef)	461	71	0.15
Chicken breast	80	360	4.50
Fast-food or frozen and breaded chicken	1,012	360	0.40
Corn (fresh)	11	219	20.00
Corn flakes	351	26	0.07
Canned corn	680	219	0.30
Shredded Wheat (Nabisco)	6	150	25.00

Table 22.1 summarizes the K-factor of some common foods. You should strive for a dietary K-factor of at least 3 and preferably higher. The K-factor of natural, unprocessed foods is quite high, as they generally contain much more potassium than sodium. The K-factor of their processed alternatives is usually too low to be healthy; processed food usually introduces a lot of sodium into the diet.

Our bodies require about 4,000 milligrams of potassium daily and can get along very well on 1,000 milligrams or less of sodium. Some low-sodium diets followed by people with high blood pressure provide no more than 500 milligrams of sodium, an amount that's quite healthy for everyone. Most diet analyses indicate that the average person gets from 7 to 10 grams of dietary sodium daily, creating a K-factor of less than 1. This explains why high blood pressure is the most widespread condition, after obesity, in the United States and most affluent countries.

Reading ingredients lists is the only way to avoid sodium in processed foods. If salt appears in the list, the food should be avoided, even if the product name or other labeling implies that it is somehow low in salt. At the bottom of the nutrition label of processed and packaged foods is a listing of the sodium and potassium content of each serving. Divide potassium by sodium to get the K-factor. Never eat a food that has a K-factor of less than 3! If the nutrition label doesn't have the sodium and potassium content, and you have the slightest doubt, avoid the product.

If you stick to natural foods, especially fruits and vegetables, you will get plenty of potassium, reduce your sodium intake, and keep a healthy dietary K-factor of greater than 3. Foods that are especially rich in potassium include bananas, artichokes, avocados, and beans. A good source of information on the amounts of sodium and potassium in foods is *Bowes & Church's Food Values of Portions Commonly Used*, by Jean A. T. Pennington, Ph.D., R.D.

To spice up foods without adding salt to your diet, try substitutes such as Tabasco sauce, horseradish, Tone Brothers Perc seasonings, and Mrs. Dash seasonings. (Tabasco sauce is high in sodium, but it is used in such small amounts—usually a drop or two—that the actual sodium consumed is insignificant.)

SODIUM AND WATER

Tap water and bottled water sometimes contain too much sodium. Often the sodium is found as salt (sodium chloride). Therefore, you must ask your municipal government about the salt content of your water. It should tell you on the label of bottled water. Do some calculations. If you drink about 64 ounces of water daily, that is a little over 2 quarts. If the water doesn't supply more than 25 milligrams of sodium per quart, it is all right. Remember, you should be drinking at least 32 ounces of water daily; it's healthy.

23

Reduce Inflammation with Omega-3 Oils

Although IBS has not been proven to be an inflammatory disease, some evidence suggests that inflammation may be involved. Inflammation involves a shift in metabolism that causes production of an excess of one prostaglandin, a hormonelike substance, over another similar prostaglandin, which increases inflammation. Many pharmaceuticals, the simplest being common aspirin, suppress production of the unwanted inflammation-causing prostaglandin. Taking aspirin or other nonsteroidal anti-inflammatory drugs (NSAIDs) for mild inflammation is commonplace nowadays. However, normal prostaglandin balance can also be achieved by diet and correct supplement use because these ingredients balance the materials from which the prostaglandins are made.

Your body produces prostaglandins from dietary oils. If we call the prostaglandin that doesn't increase inflammation the "good" prostaglandin, and the one that causes inflammation the "bad" prostaglandin, the distinction is very simple:

Good prostaglandin is produced from omega-3 oils.
Bad prostaglandin is produced from omega-6 oils.

To decrease inflammation, you'll obviously want to increase the omega-3 oils and diminish the omega-6 oils in your diet. The omega-6 oil called arachidonic acid is produced in animal tissues, so it is obtained in the diet from meat or other animal products that contain fat, such as dairy fat, eggs, and the fatty tissue in poultry. Your body can also produce it using oils found in corn oil and some other cooking and salad oils. The desired oil, eicosapentaenoic acid (EPA), is obtained from fish as well as made by the body from some vegetable sources.

Diet is essential in obtaining these oils (and is easily supported by using the correct supplements). Use olive oil on salads and for frying whenever possible and use either soy or canola oil (not other oils, such as corn oil) for other cooking because they are richer in the omega-3 oils.

For optimum prostaglandin balance, do eat:

- fish
- poultry (white meat only)
- nonfat dairy products
- vegetables and fruit
- cereals and grains
- olive oil
- canola oil
- flax oil

Don't eat:

- red meat
- dairy products that contain fat
- all processed meat, including poultry
- all corn oil products
- commercial baked goods

OMEGA-3 SUPPLEMENTS

Eicosapentaenoic Acid (EPA) Supplements

Eicosapentaenoic acid (EPA) is the critical oil for inflammation reduction and is the oil from which the good prostaglandin is made. Eicosapentaenoic acid (EPA) has been the subject of many extensive clinical studies and is safe when used sensibly and as part of a good diet. Taking up to 3 grams of EPA daily has been proven safe and effective. People with IBS, however, should start with one capsule of no more than 1,000 milligrams of EPA, taken with foods that are known not to cause an IBS flare-up. If no discomfort is experienced, you can take up to three capsules daily.

Because EPA is a fish oil, it sometimes has a somewhat fishy aftertaste. It is very unlikely this would be particularly troublesome for IBS sufferers, but it warrants careful testing to be sure. Highly purified EPA supplements are now available from which this fishy aftertaste has been removed; these are, of course, more expensive.

Flax Oil

Flax oil is about 52 percent alpha linolenic acid (ALA). ALA is converted by normal human metabolism to EPA, which is then used to make the noninflammatory prostaglandin. Years ago the human diet was quite rich in ALA and EPA from various plant sources. With the advent of corn-fattened beef and the shift away from eating green vegetables that contain omega-3 oils, dietary ALA and EPA declined. As a result, the incidence of inflammatory diseases, including multiple sclerosis, has shown an upward trend.

Flax oil is an alternative to EPA for people with IBS because the body converts it to EPA naturally; since the EPA never enters the GI tract, it can't cause any intestinal discomfort. You need to take more than 3 grams, however, because no metabolic conversion is 100 percent, and the conversion of flax oil to EPA is no different. An effective way to take flax oil is to purchase it in ½ liter (pint) bottles at your local health food store and put a tablespoonful on your food each day. Simply add a tablespoonful to your cereal each morning along with your soy milk, or add it to a salad, a baked potato, or some vegetables. Remember, however, that you cannot cook with flax oil!

Inflammation is a very complex subject, which this chapter only begins to address. For a more comprehensive discussion of inflammation, with very detailed diets, you may want to read my books, *The New Arthritis Relief Diet* and *The New Eating Right for a Bad Gut*.

24

Replenish Friendly Bacteria

An excess of unfriendly bacteria (or, more accurately, an upset in the natural microflora balance) in the large intestine will cause diarrhea. The balance is most commonly upset by food poisoning or by taking an antibiotic. Food poisoning is actually the introduction of toxic bacteria, usually salmonella, or a protozoan that upsets the normal balance. Antibiotics can cause an imbalance because they kill some bacteria and allow others to live. In either case, the natural, healthy balance is disturbed because one type of microorganism grows beyond its normal level.

Studies suggest that people with IBS have often been the victims of food poisoning from salmonella bacteria, used antibiotics extensively, or both. The illness that results from either is called *bacterial gastroenteritis*. After a bout of food poisoning or antibiotic treatment, the natural balance of healthy intestinal flora never gets reestablished, and after awhile, the symptoms become so well established that IBS is the result. The way in which IBS seems to flare up from some foods, stress, and emotional upset fits with this theory, because all those things can change the body's intestinal environment. The question then becomes, how can a person reestablish a normal intestinal microbiological balance?

You can reestablish the normal intestinal microflora by simply taking the probiotics *Lactobacillus acidophilus* and *Bifidobacteria bifidum* cultures; these should be purchased at a reputable health food store. Try to find a product that has been kept refrigerated and actually specifies the level of active bacteria on the label. The level should be at least one billion and could be as high as fifteen billion. (Don't let the numbers one billion or fifteen billion scare you. Bacteria are so small that many could get along together on the period at the end of this sentence. For your body to reestablish its normal balance, ten billion is probably about right.)

You can also purchase probiotic pills at your health food store that contain both acidophilus and bifidobacteria cultures. Always be careful to read the label in detail to be sure supplements contain live cultures. It's better if they have been refrigerated and have an expiration date. You may have to use them for a week or so before they begin to work.

YOGURT AND MILK

Some stores, including health food stores, carry yogurt and milk that contain live active acidophilus cultures. If dairy products don't trigger flare-ups for you, you can use this yogurt or milk like you would use any other milk or yogurt; for example, one serving daily.

25

Relieve Symptoms with Peppermint Oil

In Europe, enteric-coated peppermint oil is used to treat IBS. The enteric coating is resistant to digestion in both the stomach and small intestine. Once it reaches the lower intestine, however, the coating dissolves and the active peppermint is released. So do not eat peppermint candy and expect the same effect!

One clinical study showed that enteric-coated peppermint oil tablets reduced bowel frequency and all its side effects, including bloating, cramps, and flatulence. In this double-blind study, the active ingredient produced positive results about 78 percent of the time, compared to a placebo (a dummy product that looks and tastes the same but has no active ingredient), which produced results about 33 percent of the time. In most clinical studies, the placebo produces at least a 10 to 15 percent positive result. When there is a high emotional factor, such as in IBS, the placebo effect can account for as much as a 40 percent improvement.

As a result of these clinical studies, many gastroenterologists believe that peppermint oil has a definite tranquilizing effect on intestinal tissues, and therefore use the oil on the instruments that they insert through the anus into the intestine. This practice, although not based on a clinical study, is indirect support for the use of en-teric-coated peppermint oil.

Caution is essential, however. The oil must be enteric-coated. Don't purchase peppermint oil or take peppermint candy or even peppermint oil capsules and expect results; the oil must be released in the lower intestine and only enteric-coated tablets can accomplish the desired effect.

Conclusion

Having a clearly defined, non-life-threatening illness can be bad enough, but having IBS, a sort of catchall, undefinable condition, is probably worse. Thankfully, people don't die from IBS, but they must carry on with their lives as if nothing is wrong—when something most certainly is. Bowel disorders are illnesses people don't like to talk about, unlike allergies, colds, or even heart trouble or cancer. After all, who wants to chat about bowel movements? Bring the subject up too often, and you're likely to find life rather lonely.

So, people with IBS must suffer in silence, going from doctor to doctor in hopes that one will have the answer to their problem. Good luck!

As the saying goes, when you get a lemon, it's better to make lemonade than to try to swap it for an orange. When your doctor tells you that you have IBS, take the same approach. Begin by resolving that you will gain control of the condition and not allow it to prevent you from achieving your maximum potential. Start each day by taking a few moments in a quiet place, reaffirming your self-importance and your ability to achieve your goals.

Food heavily influences the intestinal environment, so you must gain control over what you eat. If you're like most people, you'll have to exchange some of your poor eating habits for better ones. Base these changes on the knowledge you gain by carefully testing your reactions to food.

Anyone with IBS must become a fiber manager as well. No matter what goes on in your digestive tract, fiber has a central role in the results. This means that you must be willing to experiment with cereals, fruits, vegetables, and fiber supplements. Each food and supplement category has many variations, so settling on the optimum combination for you will take time, patience, and perseverance. The rewards, though, will make the effort worthwhile.

Knowledge is power, in IBS as in everything else. Learn more about your genetic history; it will help you understand what challenges you face as well as what challenges might lie ahead. For example, you might learn that your problem runs in the family, but that it tends to disappear after a few years, so you can afford to be optimistic.

Finally, look in the mirror and make a self-assessment. You can't change your basic looks, but you can eliminate excess flab and strengthen muscles. Only you can decide to do so, and only you can make it happen. Again, the rewards are worth the effort. Most people who start a regular exercise program find that their bowels slowly normalize, and their IBS becomes a mere nuisance rather than a debilitating illness. You, like them, can seize control of your situation and reap the benefits!

Index

('f' indicates a figure; 't' indicates a table)